BRADY

review manual

for the EMT-Intermediate

Self-Assessment Exam Prep

BRADY

review manual

for the EMT-Intermediate

Self-Assessment Exam Prep

Joseph J. Mistovich, M. ED., NREMT-P
Department of Health Professions
Youngstown State University
Youngstown, Ohio

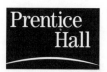
Prentice
Hall

Upper Saddle River, New Jersey 07458

Library of Congress Cataloging-in-Publication Data

Mistovich, Joseph J.
   EMT-intermediate self-assessment exam prep/Joe Mistovich
   p. cm—(Prentice Hall health review series)
   Includes index.
   ISBN 0-8359-5019-0
   1. Emergency medicine—Examinations, questions, etc. 2.
Emergency medical technicians—Examinations, questions,
etc. I. Title. II. Series.
RC86.9.M56 2001
616.02′5′076—dc21

                                           00-051644

Publisher: Julie Alexander
Executive Editor: Greg Vis
Acquisitions Editor: Katrin Beacom
Managing Development Editor: Marilyn Meserve
Director of Production and Manufacturing:
   Bruce Johnson
Managing Production Editor: Patrick Walsh
Production Editor: Jessica Balch, Pine Tree Composition
Production Liaison: Danielle Newhouse
Manufacturing Buyer: Pat Brown
Design Director: Cheryl Asherman
Design Coordinator: Maria Guglielmo
Cover and Interior Designer: Janice Bielawa
Marketing Manager: Tiffany Price
Product Information Manager: Rachele Triano
Editorial Assistant: Kierra Bloom
Composition: Pine Tree Composition
Printing and Binding: Banta Book Group

Pearson Education, Ltd., *London*
Pearson Education Australia Pty. Limited, *Sydney*
Pearson Education Singapore Pte. Ltd.
Pearson Education North Asia Ltd., *Hong Kong*
Pearson Education Canada, Ltd., *Toronto*
Pearson Educación de Mexico, S.A. de C.V.
Pearson Education—Japan, *Tokyo*
Pearson Education Malaysia, Pte. Ltd.
Pearson Education, Upper Saddle River, New Jersey

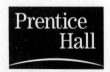

10 9 8 7 6 5 4 3 2
ISBN 0-8359-5019-0

In memory of my father, who provided me with the love and encouragement that allowed me to pursue my dreams. He will always be my inspiration to continue living life to its fullest, no matter what obstacles are encountered.

To my wife Andrea, who continues to be my biggest supporter, for her love, understanding, sincere interest in my work, and great sense of humor!

To my children, Katie, Kristyn, Chelsea, Morgan, and Kara for their unconditional love and for continuously showing me why life is so precious.

Contents

Preface

The purpose of this review manual is to help prepare you for examinations in your EMT-Intermediate course and your certification examination. The manual consists of a series of self-assessment sections that can identify your strengths and weaknesses in relation to the information you are studying. If you are a currently certified EMT-Intermediate, this manual can serve as a refresher tool itself or as a method to determine where your knowledge has deteriorated and the need for specific review.

The *EMT-Intermediate Self-Assessment Exam Prep* consists of multiple-choice type items that are organized according to the 1985 U.S. Department of Transportation's National Standard EMT-Intermediate Curriculum. Enhancement sections are included on Automated External Defibrillation, Anaphylaxis and Management, Pharmacology, and Anatomy and Physiology that are beyond the D.O.T. curriculum. Every item has a corresponding answer and rationale. In addition, every item, with the exception of those that are considered "enhancement items," is referenced to a specific D.O.T. objective, which are presented in the Appendix. These reference numbers also make it possible for you to refer back to any one of the EMT-Intermediate textbooks for more specific information on any item or overall concept.

The contributing writers all have extensive knowledge and experience as EMS educators. The items they contributed were developed in a "teacher-made test format" to allow you to test your knowledge and understanding of the material. When compiled into a series of sections, the items serve as a self-assessment tool to identify particular strengths and weakness in your knowledge and understanding of the information. This allows you to concentrate on specific sections that have been identified as a weakness.

This manual should be used as a tool to better prepare you for your examinations. However, there is no better preparation than studying and understanding the information that has been presented to you in your course. To best ensure your success on the examination, I encourage you to study first until you feel confident that you know the information, and then use this manual as a self assessment to determine how well you know the information. When you have identified areas of weakness, do not simply study the manual or review items. Go back and study the information presented to you, study the textbook, and use other sources to better understand the information. Once you again feel confident you know the material, retest yourself using the review manual to determine if you are better prepared for that section.

I hope this manual assists you in preparing for your examination. However, when it comes time to manage a patient in the prehospital environment, there is no time for preparation. You must draw on your existing knowledge and skills to successfully and efficiently treat the patient. Thus, it is imperative to good patient care that you are truly prepared not only to pass that examination but to take care of each and every patient you encounter to the best of your ability. Good luck in your EMS endeavors!

Joseph J. Mistovich

Contributors

In preparation for development of the *EMT-Intermediate Self-Assessment Exam Prep,* well-established educators were sought with years of both clinical and classroom experience. These individuals were responsible for contributing teacher-made test items based on the objectives from the U.S. Department of Transportation's National Standard EMT-Intermediate Curriculum for inclusion in this manual. The following individuals contributed a significant number of items to the *EMT-Intermediate Self-Assessment Exam Prep.*

Beth Lothrop Adams, MA, RN, NREMT-P
ALS Coordinator, EHS Programs
Adjunct Assistant Professor, Emergency Medicine
The George Washington University
Washington, D.C.

Randall W. Benner, MEd, NREMT-P
Director, Emergency Medical Technology
Instructor, Department of Health Professions
Youngstown State University
Youngstown, Ohio

Elizabeth Criss, RN, CEN, MEd
Clinical Educator, Emergency Services
Research Associate, Emergency Medicine
Arizona Health Sciences Center
Tucson, Arizona

Heather M. Drake, BS, NREMT-P
Jackson, Mississippi

James W. Drake, BS, NREMT-P
Instructor, Department of Emergency Medical Technology
University of Mississippi Medical Center
Jackson, Mississippi

Linda K. Honeycutt, EMT-P, I/C
EMS Programs Coordinator
Providence Hospital and Medical Centers
Novi, Michigan

Blaine Griffiths, BS, RN, NREMT-P
Emergency Medical Technology
Youngstown State University
Youngstown, Ohio
STAT MedEvac
Pittsburgh, Pennsylvania

Edward B. Kuvlesky, AAS, NREMT-P
President, Integrated Ideas Inc.
Battalion Chief, Indian River County EMS
Indian River County, Florida

Introduction

 SUCCESS ACROSS THE BOARDS:
THE PRENTICE HALL REVIEW SERIES

Prentice Hall is pleased to present *EMT-Intermediate Self Assessment Exam Prep* as part of a review series on the various EMS education levels. The authoritative text gives you expert help in preparing for certifying examinations.

COMPONENTS OF THE SERIES

The series is made up of a book and CD combination as well as a companion website that supports the book.

About the Book

EMT-Intermediate Self-Assessment Exam Prep by Joseph J. Mistovich: This manual has been designed to help students prepare for the written course and certification exams. It can also be used as a review for currently certified EMT-Intermediates. More than one thousand multiple-choice items are organized by the sections covered in the 1985 U.S. Department of Transportation's National Standard EMT-Intermediate Curriculum. The multiple-choice items are similar to those found on teacher-made exams and certifying exams. Working through these items will help you assess your strengths and weaknesses in each section.

- **D.O.T. Objectives:** A D.O.T objective reference number located in the answer and rationale section allows you to refer back to the specific D.O.T Curriculum objective that the item was written from. This will allow you to seek more information for each item from popular textbooks written to the D.O.T objectives. For the enhancement material that is beyond the D.O.T. objectives, answers and rationales do not have objective reference numbers. The D.O.T. objectives are presented in full in the Appendix.

- **Answers and Rationales:** Correct answers and comprehensive rationales are provided to assist you in better understanding each item. Rationales for incorrect answers are typically presented so that you may also learn why that answer is incorrect.

About the CD-ROM

A CD-ROM is included in the back of this book. It includes 200 multiple-choice questions for extra practice. A glossary of words and definitions is included to help you review the necessary terminology. In addition, for each chapter, the D.O.T. objectives covered in that particular chapter are indicated.

Companion Website for EMT-Intermediate Review

Visit the companion website at **www.brady-books.com** for additional practice, information about the exam, and links to related resources. Designed as a supplement to this book in the series, you will want to bookmark this site and return frequently for the most current information on your path to success.

STUDY TIPS

So, you're getting ready for an exam. Congratulations for making it to this point, now let's help you make the next step—doing your best on this exam. Some people find test taking unsettling, unnerving, and even scary! Use this book as an opportunity to practice physical preparation, information review, and exam techniques.

Physical Preparation

The key to maximizing your potential on a test is to be at your personal best. Along with mental preparation, physical preparation should be included in a good study strategy. Physical preparation includes getting adequate rest, and exercising. It also includes eating a balanced meal the night before and the morning of the exam. Your brain works best when it has access to supply of glucose. So fruits, grains, vegetables, and pasta are important foods. Try to avoid caffeine and foods with high sugar content on the morning of the exam. These foods provide a short burst of energy but when they are used up, the slump will significantly reduce your ability to function.

Try some physical exercise the days before the exam, although not to the point of exhaustion. Increasing cardiovascular perfusion will also increase perfusion to the brain. More oxygen circulating in the brain can only be good, right?

Exercise is also an outlet for stress, making it easier to get a good night's sleep.

Information Review

Contrary to popular belief, preparing for an exam should not include extensive last-minute studying. You've been studying for months, you know the material, and cramming now will probably cause an intellectual shutdown. Review the material for short periods of time, and take frequent breaks. Try study groups of 3–5 people for review; the active discussion will be an excellent way to reinforce the material and retain the information.

While knowing the material is essential, physical preparation is equally important. Remember, review only in brief intervals, use a study group, and don't cram.

Taking the Examination

An exam is not written by happenstance; it's an art and a science. Each time you take an exam it's a chance to evaluate your knowledge, as well as mastering the test taking process. Exams are generally built to measure *minimum* competency. Certification or recertification exams are usually not designed to test total knowledge, ability to expertly function in the field, or even your level of professionalism. They are an attempt to evaluate your reading comprehension and judgment.

There are two basic kinds of questions found on most certification exams—multiple choice and true/false. Each question is built in a specific way to test your ability and your knowledge. Knowing how the questions are constructed may help you during the exam.

Multiple choice questions consist of two parts: stems and answers. A stem is the actual question part, and the list of answers that follows contains one correct answer and several distracters. Distracters are designed to (what else?) distract you from the correct response. Multiple choice questions require you to use knowledge, judgment, and expertise in order to answer the question. *Hint:* Use the process of elimination.

When answering a multiple-choice question, read the question and all of the answers first. Then begin the process of elimination, starting with the most obvious incorrect answer and sorting your way through until you're left with one or two possible answers. Got a problem picking from those? Then re-read the stem. If it would make it easier, re-phrase the question looking for key words that give you a hint about the answer. Don't forget to look at the grammar; is the stem in plural form or singular? Whatever process you use, try not to spend more than two minutes on any one question.

You may find a topic is covered in several consecutive questions. In this case, be sure all your answers are similar and seem to fit together. It might be helpful to use the previous answers to validate each new set of choices. Another option is to check the next question because sometimes the answer, or a strong hint to one question, is the stem of the following questions. Remember, when reading multiple choice responses, the correct answer may be the most comprehensive choice—the one that combines several of the other answers or includes more details.

If the exam contains true/false questions, remember that statements containing absolute terms, like *never, always,* and *only* will usually be false. Very little of medicine, or life itself, is absolute. Statements that contain words like *maybe* or *sometimes* tend to be true.

The scientific part of test building is putting all the information into questions, and it is an art form in the way the questions are put together to evaluate you. The key is to read each question carefully—try not to scan because you miss important key words like *incorrect* or *not* which would cause you to waste time or, more important, miss the answer. Remember your all-important "three P's:" be prudent, pace yourself, and use patience.

Wrapping Up

You know how people say to go with your first hunch? Well, they're right. Your brain makes immediate connections based on stored information and your experience. Don't be afraid that the answer is wrong just because you didn't go through all the usual steps of logic. Research shows that first impressions tend to be correct.

It's okay to choose the same letter answer two or three times in a row. The answers are put into a question at random, so it could be that the same letter shows up as being correct up to five times. Don't change your answer if you have chosen the same letter more than once.

You have done the best you can by participating in class, practicing your skills, and reading your material. Trying to teach yourself the curriculum at the last minute just won't work and ultimately your patients will suffer. Trust yourself and your abilities. Practice some of the tips in this section as your proceed through this book, and in the days before the exam, remember to eat well, exercise, and get plenty of sleep.

KEYS TO SUCCESS ACROSS THE BOARDS

• Study, Review, and Practice
• Keep a positive, confident attitude
• Follow all directions on the examination
• Do your best

Good luck!

You are encouraged to visit http://www.pren-hall.com/success *for additional tips on studying, test-taking and other keys to success. At this stage of your education and career you will find these tips helpful.*

1 Roles and Responsibilities

chapter objectives

Questions in this chapter relate to DOT objectives 1.1.1–1.1.21. Please see the Appendix for more information.

DIRECTIONS Each of the questions or incomplete statements below is followed by suggested answers or completions. Select the **one answer** that is best in each case.

1. As a health care provider, the EMT-Intermediate does all of the following **except**:
   A. aims for the minimum standard of care.
   B. checks out all equipment prior to the emergency call.
   C. practices his and her skills to the point of mastery.
   D. places the patient ahead of his or her own ego.

2. Maintaining current certification is important to the EMT-Intermediate:
   A. in order to assure that patients cannot successfully sue the EMT-Intermediate.
   B. because one cannot function as an EMT-Intermediate without maintaining the requirements of certification in one's local area.
   C. to prevent being required to accrue continuing education credits.
   D. to keep malpractice insurance rates from rising.

3. All of the following are benefits of subscribing to professional journals, **except**:
   A. they are a valuable resource for current trends and latest equipment.
   B. they make the EMT-Intermediate aware of advancements in emergency medical care.
   C. they replace continuing education and/or refresher course requirements for recertification.
   D. they allow the EMT-Intermediate the opportunity to publish articles.

4. You are assessing an 88-year-old male who is complaining of head pain and numbness in his arms following a fall. The patient is in a third-floor bedroom in tight quarters. You decide it is easier to assist the patient down the stairs to the cot, instead of fully immobilizing and carrying him. Which of the following best describes this action?
   A. immoral
   B. unethical
   C. illegal
   D. incompetent

5. After checking out their ambulance in the morning, John goes to sleep on the couch. Renee notices the unit is dirty and thoroughly washes it. Which of the following best describes John's action?
   A. immoral
   B. unethical
   C. unprofessional
   D. illegal

6. The main purpose of a national association is to:
   A. promote professional development.
   B. administer national testing.
   C. establish the EMT-Intermediate curriculum.
   D. license EMT-Intermediates.

7. As an EMT-Intermediate your responsibility during an emergency response includes all of the following, **except**:
   A. size up and assure scene safety.
   B. review the call with crew members.
   C. assess the effects of treatments.
   D. maintain rapport with the patients.

8. Which of the following is **not** a responsibility of the EMT-Intermediate?

A. providing definitive emergency medical care

B. educating the public in how to recognize a medical emergency

C. instructing the public in how and when to access the EMS system

D. performing record-keeping to ensure continuity of patient care

9. Which of the following skills are included in the EMT-Intermediate training and not in the EMT-Basic?

A. administration of epinephrine for anaphylaxis

B. administration of oxygen for breathing difficulty

C. intravenous access for fluid administration

D. insertion of a nasopharyngeal airway

10. The rules and standards that govern the conduct of EMTs are referred to as:

A. morals.

B. oaths.

C. laws.

D. ethics.

11. Which of the following is **not** a professional action that should be displayed by the EMT-Intermediate?

A. Performing skills at a minimally acceptable level

B. Critically reviewing your performance looking for areas to refine

C. Setting high standards for yourself, your crew and your system

D. Understanding the importance of response times

12. Which of the following statements about continuing education is **true**?

A. The goal is to review previously learned material and receive new information.

B. Continuing education is not necessary after certification or licensure.

C. Graduating from an EMT-Intermediate program assures the public of quality patient care.

D. As the volume of calls decrease, training should also decrease.

13. The standards of conduct or rules that influence a particular group are known as:

A. group dynamics.

B. group morality.

C. group responsibility.

D. ethics.

14. The qualities, conduct, and actions that portray emergency medical service personnel are called:

A. practical training.

B. professionalism.

C. professional development.

D. educational development.

15. You suspect that your partner is stealing prescription medications from patients you have transported. You have no specific evidence to prove your suspicions. In regard to your position in this matter, this is an example of a(n):

A. ethical (moral) dilemma.

B. legal dilemma.

C. operational dilemma.

D. institutional dilemma.

16. You observe a co-worker stealing from a patient's home. In regard to your position in this matter, this is an example of a(n):

A. legal dilemma.

B. institutional dilemma.

C. operational dilemma.

D. ethical (moral) dilemma.

17. Continuing education is important for all of the following reasons, **except**:
    A. it provides a method of obtaining new knowledge and skills.
    B. it prevents decay of skill competency.
    C. it is an opportunity to learn basic skills that you have not become proficient in.
    D. it reinforces current treatment practices.

18. The process by which a governmental agency provides permission to an EMT-I to function is called:
    A. licensure or certification.
    B. registration.
    C. protocol or standing orders.
    D. credentialing.

19. Select the statement that best describes the term **professional**.
    A. Driven by ego, this individual is confident in the durability of his/her skills and knowledge.
    B. This person practices skills to the point of mastery and continually seeks opportunities to increase knowledge and skills.
    C. This individual aims to meet minimum standards, relies on others to check and maintain equipment and supplies.
    D. This individual resents evaluations or run reviews and blames others for own inadequacies.

20. Continuing education is important for all of the following reasons, **except**:
    A. infrequent use causes skills and knowledge to suffer.
    B. it reviews previous learning and provides new information.
    C. training should increase with an increase in call volume.
    D. everyone experiences a decay in skills and knowledge.

21. The major purposes of a national registration agency are:
    A. to provide verification of training through a standardized exam process and set a standard for evaluating competency.
    B. to limit the number of nationally certified EMT-Intermediates and establish a national minimum standard of care.
    C. to establish a limited number of training programs that meet a national standard and to administer standardized exams.
    D. to establish qualifications for registration and to publish a journal to fulfill continuing education requirements.

22. While transporting a burn patient to the hospital, the receiving physician requests that you administer morphine for pain relief. Since you already have established an IV, you should:
    A. request the amount of morphine to administer.
    B. request that the physician reverify the drug order.
    C. state that administering morphine is beyond your scope of practice.
    D. state that you will administer it if he or she grants you special permission.

23. The most important action an EMT-I could take personally which would increase the public's awareness about automated external defibrillation in cases of cardiac arrest, is:
    A. tell the public relations officer.
    B. tell his or her field supervisor.
    C. consider speaking at local public events.
    D. pay for advertisements which will appear in local newspapers.

24. All of the following are acceptable practices for the EMT-Intermediate, **except**:
    A. administering electrical shocks for ventricular fibrillation.

B. initiating an IV for a multisystem trauma patient.

C. applying oxygen for a COPD patient.

D. administering Mannitol to a head injured patient.

Questions 25 and 26 refer to the following information:

You are called to treat a gunman who was shot by police after assaulting an elderly woman and her young granddaughter. The patient suffers an unexpected cardiac arrest in your care.

25. Based on this scenario, choose the statement below which is most correct.
   A. Failure to treat the patient to the best of your ability violates the Fair Treatment Act.
   B. Neglecting to treat the patient appropriately is considered illegal.
   C. Neglecting to treat the patient appropriately can make you liable for his death.
   D. None of the above are correct.

26. Your failure to treat the gunman appropriately may also be considered:
   A. unethical.
   B. legal.
   C. appropriate.
   D. righteous.

27. The best method to ensure that you are acting ethically is to:
   A. know the laws governing EMS in your state.
   B. avoid performing illegal acts while providing care.
   C. place the patient's welfare above everything but your own safety.

D. become emotionally attached to each patient as if he or she was a member of your own family.

28. You have just completed a long-distance transfer of a patient to a hospital in another state. You have just left the hospital when you come across a woman standing at the curb who is feverishly waving you down. You stop your ambulance and get out and find an elderly man on the front lawn in cardiac arrest. You get your equipment out of the ambulance and begin resuscitation, including defibrillation and IV therapy. Your act of resuscitating this patient would be considered:
   A. illegal and unethical.
   B. illegal but ethical.
   C. legal and ethical.
   D. legal but unethical.

29. While at the scene of a mass casualty, an EMT-Intermediate refuses to serve as the communications officer because he wants to be where the action is. His behavior would be considered:
   A. unethical.
   B. illegal.
   C. unprofessional.
   D. respectful.

30. Your partner states that his EMT-Intermediate card expired two weeks ago. However, he continues to function without telling his superiors that his certification has lapsed because he really needs the money and his family can't afford to go without a paycheck. Your partner's act is:
   A. illegal.
   B. ethical.
   C. professional.
   D. justifiable.

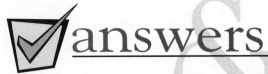answers
& rationales

1.

A. Professionals set high standards for themselves, their crew, their agency, and their system. Non-professionals aim for minimum standards. *(1.1.10)*

2.

B. The EMT-Intermediate needs to keep certification current to remain employed. By maintaining certification, the public can be assured the EMT-Intermediate has fulfilled all continuing education requirements deemed necessary by the state and/or local jurisdiction. *(1.1.17)*

3.

C. Professional journals keep the EMT-Intermediate abreast of the latest changes in an ever-changing industry. These journals provide an abundant source of continuing education material, as well as an excellent opportunity for EMS professionals to write and publish articles. However, the journals do not replace the need for continuing education and refresher courses. *(1.1.20)*

4.

B. The EMT code of ethics states that as a health care professional, the EMT should "do no harm." In this case, the patient is symptomatic of a spinal injury secondary to a fall. Subsequently, he requires full immobilization in an attempt to avoid worsening the injury. Ethics govern behavior in terms of right or wrong. Failure to fully immobilize this patient could worsen an existing injury and would be considered wrong from the standpoint of "do no harm." Therefore, this action would be unethical. *(1.1.8)*

5.

C. True professionalism is not given but earned. Professionals in EMS constantly strive to promote high standards and instill pride in their profession. By washing the dirty ambulance, Renee is accomplishing just that. Ethics and morals do not apply here in that washing the ambulance cannot be said to be right or wrong and has little to do with the actual patient care given by the pair. *(1.1.12)*

6.

A. National associations strive to promote professional development by offering educational opportunities and instilling individual awareness of the need for continual self-improvement. National associations do not conduct national testing, establish curriculum, or license EMT-Intermediates; these are generally left up to national registration agencies and/or individual states. *(1.1.18)*

7.

B. Reviewing (critiquing) the call with crew members will improve future team performance, however, this is not a part of your emergency response duties. This should be done after the response. *(1.1.2)*

8.

A. The medical director is ultimately responsible for all patient care. The EMT-Intermediate legally functions at the discretion of the medical director. Providing definitive care is not a function of the EMT-Intermediate and is conducted by the medical staff at the receiving hospital or health care facility. *(1.1.2)*

9.

C. Intravenous access is a skill taught to EMT-Intermediates and not EMT-Basics. EMT-Basics under the 1994 U.S. Department of Transportation curriculum can assist with the administration of epinephrine in anaphylaxis. The administration of oxygen and insertion of a nasophayrngeal airway have been standard practices for EMT-Basics for several years. *(1.1.3)*

10.

D. Ethics are the rules or standards that govern the conduct of members of a particular group. Furthermore, they set standards of right or wrong for humane conduct. Laws and regulations will obligate you to follow certain actions and are bound by statutes. *(1.1.5)*

11.

A. Skills performed by an EMT-Intermediate must be mastered. Attaining and maintaining skills at a minimally acceptable level is not considered a professional attribute. The professional masters the skills and continuously practices them to keep them from deteriorating to a substandard level. *(1.1.12)*

12.

A. You should constantly review previously learned material, as well as attain new information. Certification or licensure marks only the beginning of your lifelong learning process. Continuing education and recertification requirements will contribute to quality patient care. Merely graduating from a training program does not ensure long-term quality. When the volume of calls decrease, the continuing education requirements must increase to compensate for the reduction in skill performance. *(1.1.13)*

13.

D. Ethics is the study of actions that govern group behavior. What action is "right or "wrong" within a group? The group determines "standards of conduct" called ethics. Although ethics are not laws, most laws have an ethical foundation. When dealing with difficult ethical situations, it is always best to do what is in the patient's best interest. *(1.1.4)*

14.

B. Professionalism is displayed by qualities and conduct in persons such as the promotion of quality health care, pride in their profession, and setting high goals for themselves. Other members of the health care team respect and have confidence in the professional's abilities. Professionalism requires the paramedic to strive to high levels of performance and communication. *(1.1.4)*

15.

A. This is an example of an ethical (moral) dilemma or problem. There is not enough "evidence" to make this incident a legal issue. This situation certainly creates an ethical dilemma for you. Do you report your suspicions to your employer? Do you talk with your partner about your suspicions? Or, do you say nothing? This is a classic example of an ethical decision that you may be forced to make during your career. *(1.1.5)*

16.

A. This is an example of a legal dilemma or issue. You actually witnessed your partner performing an illegal act, which requires you to report the incident immediately to the proper authorities. Ethically and legally, stealing is wrong. *(1.1.5)*

17.

C. Continuing education is not designed to replace the knowledge base and skill competence attained during your initial training program. You should be proficient in all skills before receiving certification or licensure as an EMT-Intermediate. Patients should not be your tool to practice to become competent; however, patients will keep your skills current. *(1.1.14)*

18.

A. Licensure or certification is a process that grants an individual formal permission to engage in a specific occupation. Registration provides recognition that an individual has met certain qualifications. This is usually performed by a governmental or private agency. *(1.1.15)*

19.

B. A professional is an individual whose conduct characterizes a practitioner in a particular filed. It is not a matter of pay; it is attitude. The EMS professional is someone who establishes excellence as a goal and continually works to improve his/her skills and knowledge in order to provide the best patient care possible. *(1.1.9)*

20.

C. Continuing education is important for all EMT-Intermediates because infrequent use causes skills and knowledge to suffer. It reviews previous learning and provides new information. Everyone experiences decay in skills and knowledge. Typically, training should increase with a decrease in call volume. *(1.1.14)*

21.

A. The major purposes of a national registration agency are to provide verification of training through a standardized exam process and set a standard for evaluating competency. *(1.1.19)*

22.

C. Administration of morphine is a skill which is beyond the scope of practice for an EMT-I. Specifically, morphine can only be administered by an EMT-Paramedic in the prehospital environment. Therefore requesting special permission and asking for the dose are irrelevant since the EMT-I cannot administer it anyway. *(1.1.1)*

23.

C. Prehospital care providers are often called upon to use their knowledge in helping the public become more aware of emergency medical services. Commonly, they also help with courses such as CPR and first aid. Notifying your supervisor, public relations officer, or placing newspaper ads are options, however, providing public education through personal appearances at meetings is the best option. *(1.1.21)*

24.

D. There are numerous skills taught to prehospital care providers in order to effectively treat patients. It is very important, however, to know exactly what you can or cannot do at the EMT-I level. Defibrillation, oxygen administration, and IV initiation are all acceptable skills for the EMT-I. Administering Mannitol for a head injured patient, according to the U.S. Department of Transportation's National Standard EMT-Intermediate Curriculum, is not. *(1.1.16)*

25.

C. Regardless of your impression of the patient as a person or as a member of society, you cannot allow your prejudices or opinions to influence your care. As such, failure to treat the patient to the best of your ability can make you liable for his death. The Fair Treatment Act has nothing to do with prehospital care, and the degree of legality in not following standing orders for treatment is not the cause of your liability. *(1.1.7)*

26.

A. Not treating him to the best of your ability because you have developed an opinion about him is considered unethical. EMTs cannot prejudge patients. Following your protocols and treating the patient to the best of your ability will be deemed appropriate, legal, and ethical. *(1.1.8)*

27.

C. Ethical activity involves placing the patient's welfare above everything but your own safety. Knowing the laws of your state may prevent you from performing illegal acts, but not necessarily unethical acts. As an EMT-I, you must not become emotionally attached to your patient, however maintain a detached concern for him or her. *(1.1.6)*

28.

B. Stopping and assisting the elderly man is considered ethical behavior. However, providing care at an advanced level out of your certification or licensure jurisdiction, in this case another state, is considered illegal. *(1.1.7)*

29.

C. Refusing to serve as the communications officer is an unprofessional act. It does not constitute illegal or unethical behavior since he is not refusing to deliver care to the injured patients. *(1.1.11)*

30.

A. It is imperative to keep your certification or license current while practicing prehospital care. If your certification or license should lapse and you continue to function as an EMT-Intermediate, you are acting illegally. It is your legal, ethical, and professional responsibility to keep your certifications and licensure current. *(1.1.17)*

2 EMS Systems

chapter objectives

Questions in this chapter relate to DOT objectives 1.2.1–1.2.23. Please see the Appendix for more information.

DIRECTIONS Each of the questions or incomplete statements below is followed by suggested answers or completions. Select the **one answer** that is best in each case.

1. You are treating a major trauma patient with suspected internal bleeding. What is your major goal for this patient's care?
   A. Wait for the paramedic backup to arrive because you can do nothing for this patient.
   B. Spend as much time as possible on the scene to get a complete, accurate description of the whole accident scene.
   C. Initiate treatment for this patient, including immobilization, oxygen therapy, and fluid therapy, with rapid transport to the appropriate facility.
   D. Transport this patient, as rapidly as possible to the closest trauma center.

2. How would you best describe protocols?
   A. Protocols allow you to treat the patient any way you deem necessary.
   B. Protocols are suggestions of how you could possibly treat your patient.
   C. Protocols are sets of policies that only paramedics follow, so they are not important to you as an EMT-Intermediate.
   D. Protocols are guidelines that provide a standardized emergency care plan for patient treatment.

3. What is your most important responsibility once you arrive at the receiving facility?
   A. To complete a prehospital care report.
   B. To drop off the patient so you can get ready for your next call.
   C. To relay patient information to the first orderly you see.
   D. Transfer the care of the patient to appropriate medical personnel and relay the patient information and treatment.

4. Which one of the following patient conditions could be most definitively treated in the prehospital environment prior to transport?
   A. hypoglycemia
   B. cardiac arrest
   C. drug overdose
   D. stroke

5. Of the following, which organization has the greatest influence over EMS training standards?
   A. the National Registry of EMTs
   B. the American Ambulance Association
   C. the state EMS office
   D. the regional EMS committee

6. Under which emergency situation should you be most concerned with transport time to the hospital?
   A. an unresponsive patient from an overdose
   B. an unresponsive patient with blunt abdominal trauma
   C. a responsive patient complaining of chest pain
   D. a responsive patient with an open tibia fracture

7. You have initiated an IV on an alert and oriented 38-year-old male whose chief complaint is general malaise. The patient informs you that he wishes to be transported to a facility where his family doctor is located. However, this facility is out of your jurisdiction. What would be the best way to handle this situation?

   A. Transport the patient to the out of jurisdiction facility.

   B. Transport the patient to a local facility because of the initiation of the IV.

   C. Contact the patient's family doctor for permission to transport to requested hospital.

   D. Contact the medical control physician for advice.

8. Earlier in the day you transported an unresponsive female patient to a local facility for hyperpyrexia. During dinner, you suddenly realize that you did not inform the emergency department staff that the patient was on Coumadin. What would you do in this situation?

   A. No action is necessary because the medication has nothing to do with hyperpyrexia.

   B. Inform the emergency department physician immediately.

   C. Inform the emergency department ward clerk.

   D. Your written documentation will adequately cover this omission.

9. Returning from lunch, you and your partner come across a vehicle that has sheared a utility pole. On the roadway, there is one patient next to the car. The patient appears severely dyspneic with an active arterial bleed from the left thigh. What would be your initial action?

   A. control the major bleeding

   B. perform a scene size-up

   C. establish and maintain an airway

   D. stabilize the vehicle

10. Of the following people, who decides who can provide care for patients within an EMS system?

   A. EMT supervisor

   B. EMS administrator

   C. medical director

   D. senior paramedic

11. Which of the following best describes on-line medical control?

   A. Prehospital providers communicate by radio with a physician regarding patient treatment.

   B. Prehospital providers follow written protocols.

   C. Prehospital providers communicate with the emergency department's staff to notify them of the patient's arrival.

   D. Prehospital providers notify the physician of this patient's condition while en route to the emergency department.

12. Which of the following is not a skill that would be performed by an EMT-Intermediate?

   A. hemorrhage control

   B. needle cricothyrotomy

   C. intravenous fluid therapy

   D. fluid bolus therapy

13. An EMS quality assurance (QA) program is best described by which of the following?

   A. occasional monitoring and measurement of the quality of medical care being delivered

   B. continuous monitoring and measurement of the quality of clinical care delivered

   C. a measurable means of focusing on customer perceptions of the service provided

   D. refining the system in an attempt to provide the quickest response times

14. Because the nursing staff at the hospital is busy, you provide the oral report to and transfer care to a nurse's aide. This action may be interpreted as:
    A. assault.
    B. criminal malfeasance.
    C. negligence.
    D. abandonment.

15. A program that provides physician reviews and critiques of run reports for the purpose of refining the EMS system and improving patient care is known as:
    A. protocol disciplinary.
    B. quality assurance.
    C. negligence reduction.
    D. risk management.

16. A man tells you he is a physician and questions the treatment you are providing. The man asks you to perform and administer a larger dose of a drug that you consider to be inappropriate. You should:
    A. ask that the medical control physician's authority be transferred to the on-scene physician.
    B. deny any orders and contact the medical control physician for patient care authority.
    C. ask that the medical control physician's authority be transferred to the on-scene physician if proper identification is provided.
    D. if unsure, make all management decisions with input from both physicians.

17. Federal specifications for ambulance design developed by the Government Services Administration are called the:
    A. BLS-GSA standards.
    B. EMS-A standards.
    C. ALS 1822 standards.
    D. KKK-A-1822 standards.

18. A recommended list of equipment that should be carried on Basic Life Support units was established in 1983 by the:
    A. National Association of Emergency Medical Technicians.
    B. American College of Emergency Physicians.
    C. American Medical Association.
    D. American College of Surgeon's Committee on Trauma.

19. Guidelines that are used when providing emergency care are called:
    A. protocol.
    B. emergency care standards.
    C. treatment management plan.
    D. on-line orders.

20. Which statement best describes the relationship between the EMT-Intermediate and the medical control physician?
    A. The EMT-Intermediate functions independently on his own certification or license.
    B. Care provided is solely the responsibility of the physician.
    C. The physician provides the legal right for the EMT-I to function.
    D. The responsibility for care provided rests solely with the EMT-Intermediate.

21. Which general statement best describes the difference in the prehospital management of trauma versus medical patients?
    A. Trauma patients require rapid transport; medical patients are typically transported after stabilization.
    B. Medical patients require rapid transport; trauma patients are transported after stabilization.
    C. All trauma and medical patients are transported rapidly.
    D. All trauma and medical patients are stabilized prior to transport.

22. To be effective, medical control must have official and clearly defined authority over all aspects of the delivery of prehospital emergency care because:
    A. Protocols cannot be developed to cover every possible emergency situation.
    B. Public safety can only be assured if EMS providers receive close supervision.
    C. Very few who require assistance from EMS are found in situations where a physician is present.
    D. All prehospital care provided is done so under the medical director's control.

23. State laws affect many aspects of the delivery of prehosptial emergency care including:
    A. scope of practice.
    B. third-party billing.
    C. scheduling practices.
    D. direct budget control.

24. Communication with a base hospital physician for treatment orders is also known as:
    A. off-line medical control.
    B. physician-directed care.
    C. on-line medical control.
    D. standing orders.

25. Which of the following should be the priority upon arrival at a car crash?
    A. Ascertain if the patient is conscious or unconscious.
    B. Assess the patient for possible life threats.
    C. Examine the scene for hazards.
    D. Determine if the fire department can gain access into the vehicle.

26. An example of an off-line order is:
    A. initiating an IV line on a trauma patient prior to reporting the condition to the physician.
    B. contacting the medical control and asking permission to initiate the trauma protocol.

    C. requesting a trauma team on a patient involved in a shooting.
    D. contacting dispatch for a helicopter for medical evacuation.

27. What should you do when a physician on-scene orders you to administer medication not included in your protocol?
    A. Follow the on-scene physician's order as long as he signs your EMS report.
    B. Have the on-scene physician speak with your medical control regarding patient care.
    C. Instruct the on-scene physician to leave the scene or be arrested.
    D. Ask the physician to provide proof of his identity.

28. Development of treatment protocols should be guided by all of the following except:
    A. the EMS director(s) and provider.
    B. state laws.
    C. the medical director(s).
    D. billing department.

29. An enhanced 9-1-1 system:
    A. provides the caller's phone number, and location.
    B. provides only a call-back number.
    C. always identifies the caller's name.
    D. is nothing more than a call forwarding system.

30. Earlier in the shift you transported a 58-year-old male patient with chest pain. Later that day you take another patient to the same emergency department. While there you inquire about the diagnosis and condition of the 58-year-old chest pain patient, since both you and your partner did not believe the chest pain was caused by a myocardial infarction. Your activity is considered:

A. to be a method of performing quality assurance and continuous quality improvement.

B. illegal and unethical.

C. unprofessional since you are not permitted to discuss the case of another patient.

D. to be a breach of the laws of confidentiality.

31. Which of the following best describes your responsibilities once you have delivered the patient to the emergency department?

A. You are not responsible for the patient once you are in the emergency department.

B. It is necessary that you provide an oral and written report to ensure a continuum of care in the emergency department.

C. You do not need to provide an oral report to the emergency department staff since all the information will be contained within your EMS report.

D. It is not necessary to report any additional findings while en route to the hospital because the physician will conduct his own physical exam on the patient.

32. Ideally, equipment and supplies that are used on a call should be replaced:

A. at the end of the shift.

B. by the next crew coming on duty.

C. by the supply officer who checks the ambulance at the beginning of the shift.

D. immediately after transferring patient care to the emergency department and prior to going back into service.

33. Which of the following would be an example of a non-clinical continuous quality improvement system evaluation tool?

A. a review of the EMS report for proper documentation of patient medications

B. a run review conducted by the local EMS physician director

C. a survey sent to a patient regarding your appearance at the scene

D. a report written by the emergency department nurse indicating the excessive number of IV attempts on one patient

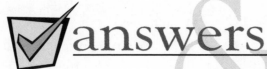

answers & rationales

1.

C. While some information is needed about the accident scene, the major goal should be initiating treatment and stabilizing the patient as an extension of the hospital environment. Severe trauma patients need rapid transport for further care and access to an operating room. However, initial treatment to manage immediate life threats should be performed. Valuable time should not be spent acquiring a complete accident profile. *(1.2.2)*

2.

D. Protocols are important for the EMT-Intermediate. They provide a basis for medical care and a standardized approach to the patient. *(1.2.13)*

3.

D. Your responsibility to your patient does not end until you transfer care to appropriate medical personnel (doctor or nurse) at the hospital. The EMT-Intermediate must report the patient's status, the treatment that was initiated, and any response to the prehospital treatment. *(1.2.21)*

4.

A. Definitive patient care must be provided as soon as possible. For some patients this can be started and, to a great measure, completed in the field. While all these patients require transport to the hospital, a hypoglycemic may be treated in the field with oral glucose or 50% Dextrose IV. The other three patients could receive initial prehospital stabilization, and then definitive treatment in-hospital. *(1.2.3)*

5.

C. Your state EMS office provides legal requirements on training standards that must be adhered to. The National Registry of EMTs is an organization designed to provide only testing to EMS personnel. The American Ambulance Association provides a forum to EMS agencies. *(1.2.14)*

6.

B. Certain prehospital emergencies, specifically trauma, can only be managed in the hospital's emergency department or operating suite. As such, resuscitation measures for major trauma patients must be initiated in the field or during transport with rapid movement of the patient to an appropriate medical facility. Recognizing the differing philosophies between treating medical and trauma patients in the prehospital environment by the EMT-Intermediate is pivotal in decreasing morbidity and mortality from trauma. *(1.2.20)*

7.

D. Contact the medical control physician for advice. As an EMT-Intermediate you practice under the control of the medical director who has delegated authority to other medical control physicians. Therefore, you must contact the medical control physician for advice and permission to transport this patient to another facility. Transporting this patient to the out-of-jurisdiction facility without the advisement of medical control would be a blatant violation of the physician/EMT-Intermediate relationship—especially if something detrimental happened en route. Transporting the patient to the local facility may be unnecessary depending upon the decision of the medical control physician. In this situation, you are not accountable to the family doctor. *(1.2.5)*

8.

B. The patient care continuum begins when treatment is initiated in the field and extends into the emergency department. This continuum is made possible by effective communication between prehospital personnel and the emergency department staff. Failure to communicate breaks this continuum and ultimately compromises patient care. The omission in relaying the medication history can affect the way a patient is treated or evaluated in the emergency department and quite possibly ultimate patient outcome. The emergency department physician is directly responsible for the general welfare of the patient. In this sense, merely contacting the emergency department clerk is not the best selection. Direct communication with the emergency department physician would be the best way to resolve this oversight. *(1.2.16)*

9.

B. Your initial responsibility on the scene lies in sizing up the incident, determining what resources will be needed, and assuring that the scene is safe prior to entry. In this situation, you must locate any potential hazards and identify the number and severity of patients so additional resources can be dispatched. *(1.2.18)*

10.

C. The EMS system must retain a medical director. The medical director provides the legal right for an EMT-Intermediate to function. *(1.2.4)*

11.

A. On-line medical control requires you to communicate directly with the physician by radio, phone, or other communicating devices. *(1.2.5)*

12.

B. Performing a needle cricothyrotomy is a paramedic skill. *(1.2.10)*

13.

B. A quality-assurance program is typically designed to point out the problems that a system may experience. This is often done through a continuing education process. A continuous quality improvement (CQI) program is committed to improving the whole system through customer perception and focuses on recognizing and rewarding good performances instead of pointing out the problems. *(1.2.11)*

14.

D. Anytime you relinquish patient care to personnel with less training than yourself you are abandoning your patient. Negligence is a deviation from accepted standards of care recognized by law. *(1.2.21)*

15.

B. Quality assurance programs may include physician review of run reports. Evaluation of such data may include response times, adherence to protocols, and other trends that may improve the patient service. *(1.2.22)*

16.

B. In this scenario, care and direct communication with the medical control physician is imperative. The management decisions are to be provided by the medical control physician. If care is provided by a physician prior to arrival of the EMT-Intermediate and medical control communications are not established, do the following: Make sure you look at proper identification. Ensure that the physician will accept responsibility and document the care as required by the local system. If the treatment is different than that established by the system, the physician should accompany (in the ambulance) the patient to the hospital. If the physician does not agree to these terms, the medical control physician regains responsibility for patient care. *(1.2.6)*

17.

D. In 1974, the Department of Transportation asked the Federal General Services Administration to develop specifications for ambulances. This goal was to standardize ambulance design and construction. Currently design and construction standards exist on three types of ambulances: Types I, II, and III. *(1.2.8)*

18.

D. The recommended Basic Life Support equipment and supplies list was developed by the American College of Surgeons, Committee on Trauma. In 1988 the American College of Emergency Physician's published a list of advanced life support equipment and supplies that should be carried on Advanced Life Support units. Most state laws governing EMS systems use these lists. They act as a guide for the development of state required equipment and supplies. *(1.2.9)*

19.

B. Protocols provide guidelines that facilitate delivery of emergency care. Standing orders allow specific interventions to be carried out without direct medical control. Usually standing orders describe the specific delivery of emergency care. The protocol could include off-line orders that are written standard or on-line orders that require you to contact medical control for permission to perform specific care. Standing orders are used when medical control cannot be contacted. *(1.2.12)*

20.

C. EMT-Intermediate's legal right to function is derived from medical control physician. Care provided by the EMT-Intermediate is considered an extension of the medical control physician. In practice, the responsibilities are shared. *(1.2.19)*

21.

A. The critical trauma patient requires rapid transport. Surgery is often required to manage the trauma patient's condition. The quicker the patient's traumatic injury is identified and bleeding is stopped, the greater the chance the patient will survive. In general, medical patients are typically provided more on-scene stabilization prior to transport. Not all patients are transported rapidly and all patients are not stabilized prior to transport. *(1.2.20)*

22.

D. All prehospital care provided is done so under the medical director's authority. Therefore, in order to be effective, medical control must have official and clearly defined authority over all aspects of the delivery of prehospital emergency care. *(1.2.4)*

23.

A. Legislation affects many aspects of the delivery of prehospital medical care including the scope of practice. Motor vehicle laws governing the operation of emergency vehicles and Good Samaritan Laws are also addressed. *(1.2.15)*

24.

C. Direct communication with a base hospital physician for treatment orders during an emergency call is known as on-line medical control. *(1.2.19)*

25.

C. All the answers listed must be accomplished by the EMT-I on the scene of a car crash. The order, however, is important. The first thing that must be done is assuring the safety of you and your crew, as well as other rescue personnel. *(1.2.18)*

26.

A. Protocols and standing orders are the guidelines provided by the medical director governing patient care. If you carry out treatment based on written guidelines, it is an example of off-line medical direction. If the protocol requires you to first consult the medical director prior to providing care, this is an example of on-line medical control. Initiating an IV line prior to physician contact would be an off-line order. *(1.2.12)*

27.

B. Whenever a physician is on-scene and wants to influence your treatment, it is best to have that physician speak directly to the medical control physician regarding patient care options. This is done so that optimal patient care can be discussed between the physicians (often the on-scene physician does not know your standing orders). The on-scene physician must also agree to travel with you to the hospital in the ambulance if he or she decides to assume responsibility for patient care and continue to direct patient care. *(1.2.6)*

28.

D. All the named individuals should be part of the decision making process in development or revision of standing orders except for the billing department. The medical aspect of the provision of emergency medical services is not influenced by the billing department or any insurance providers. *(1.2.13)*

29.

A. An enhanced 9-1-1 system is ideal because it automatically provides a phone number (ANI) and location (ALI) information. Therefore, the 9-1-1 call taker has a callback number and location of the caller immediately upon answering the line. The caller's name is provided for residential lines, however, pay phones only provide location and number. *(1.2.1)*

30.

A. One method of continuous quality improvement that EMT-Is are encouraged to perform is a follow-up on the patients that they have treated. You can com-

pare your field impression with the official diagnosis and determine if your field treatment was correct and accurate. This is not a breach of confidentially since it involves the patient that you cared for and transported. *(1.2.7)*

31.

B. Your care for the patient does not stop when you step foot into the emergency department. An orderly transfer of care must be established so that the continuum of care from the prehospital setting to the hospital environment is ensured. Both your oral and written reports are important in establishing the continuum of care for the patient. Leaving the patient in the emergency department without a proper transfer of care to an equally- or higher-trained medical professional may constitute abandonment. *(1.2.16)*

32.

D. Ideally, all equipment and supplies should be replenished immediately after each call. This would enable you to go back into service with a fully stocked and ready ambulance. *(1.2.17)*

33.

C. Continuous quality improvement systems look at both clinical and non-clinical aspects of the EMS system. Non-clinical aspects may include billing, maintenance, and supply. Your appearance and professionalism may also be assessed. *(1.2.23)*

3 Medical/Legal Considerations

chapter objectives

Questions in this chapter relate to DOT objectives 1.3.1–1.3.7. Please see the Appendix for more information.

DIRECTIONS Each of the questions or incomplete statements below is followed by suggested answers or completions. Select the **one answer** that is best in each case.

1. A patient is made aware of the benefits and risks of emergency medical care, and agrees to such treatment. The patient has provided what type of consent?
   A. implied
   B. informed
   C. emancipated
   D. rational

2. You and your partner are treating a 57-year-old male who is complaining of difficulty breathing. You have the patient on a non-rebreather mask at 15 lpm, and NS running at TKO. En route to the hospital, you pass a motor vehicle accident where a BLS unit is on-scene and has requested your assistance for their critical patient. You have the BLS crew transport your patient, while you provide emergency care to the trauma patient. Your action can be considered to be:
   A. ethical.
   B. failure of duty to act.
   C. proximate cause treatment.
   D. abandonment.

3. In order to determine that the EMT-Intermediate is negligent, all of the following elements must be proven, **except**:
   A. medical control was contacted.
   B. the injury that occurred was a direct result of the EMT-Intermediate's action or inaction.
   C. injury to the patient resulted.
   D. the EMT-Intermediate had a duty to act and breached that duty.

4. You are treating a 14-year-old boy with evidence of abdominal trauma and a tender rigid abdomen. Currently, he is alert and oriented and is refusing treatment and transport. The boy's 16-year-old brother states that his parents are at work and would not want him treated. You should:
   A. provide emergency care and transport the patient.
   B. have the patient sign a refusal form and leave the scene.
   C. have the brother transport the patient.
   D. contact the parents for permission to provide emergency care.

5. Your threat that your patient is going to get an IV whether he wants one or not would constitute:
   A. slander.
   B. assault.
   C. battery.
   D. libel.

6. You are called to the scene of an attempted suicide and find a behaviorally unstable and violent patient who is a potential threat to himself and others. Medical direction has indicated it is necessary to transport the patient. How should you best respond to the situation?
   A. Contact medical control for an order for a sedative.
   B. Restrain the patient by using whatever means necessary.
   C. Use reasonable force to secure the patient.
   D. Leave the scene.

7. You have decided to provide positive pressure ventilation (PPV) to a COPD patient who is conscious, but in acute respiratory failure. You attempt to explain the procedure to the patient in order to obtain consent, but the patient does not seem to fully understand. You should:

   A. continue emergency care and provide the positive pressure ventilation.

   B. stop emergency care until you get verbal consent.

   C. gain expressed consent prior to any invasive procedures.

   D. Informed consent is not necessary or applied to emergency medical care.

8. Which of the following best illustrates the concept of an act of libel?

   A. Writing, "This patient is a drunk," on your EMS run report.

   B. Saying, "This patient is a drunk," to the ED physician.

   C. Writing, "This patient claims she was raped," on your EMS run report.

   D. Saying, "This patient claims she was raped," to the ED physician.

9. Which one of the following charges may result if you fail to obtain expressed consent prior to initiating care?

   A. abandonment

   B. false imprisonment

   C. assault and battery

   D. slander

10. A 72-year-old female who is alert and oriented complains of dizziness. She refuses all interventions aside from transport. After she is strapped to the cot, you put a nasal cannula on her as per your protocol. She becomes very agitated. Your action is best described as:

    A. justifiable per protocol.

    B. legal via involuntary consent.

    C. a form of false imprisonment.

    D. illegal under these circumstances.

11. You make contact with a 62-year-old male whose level of consciousness is decreased. You state your name, title, and ask him if he wishes you to help him. He moans and nods his head. What type of consent have you obtained?

    A. no consent

    B. implied consent

    C. informed consent

    D. expressed consent

12. You arrive at a one-car crash. The driver of the vehicle is sitting about 20 feet away from the car on a grassy patch. Which of the following statements would be a priority in the written documentation about this incident?

    A. Patient self-extricated himself from the vehicle.

    B. Patient is intoxicated.

    C. Firearm found on the front passenger seat.

    D. Patient making derogatory remarks toward the EMS crew.

13. Which of the following best describes the state's legislation that defines the scope and role of the EMT-Intermediate?

    A. National Practitioner Act

    B. Good Samaritan Laws

    C. Delegation of Authority Act

    D. State Medical Practice Act

14. The patient you are assessing is alert but responding inappropriately. You should:

    A. begin emergency care per your protocol.

    B. attempt to gain expressed consent.

    C. use involuntary consent to provide care.

    D. wait several minutes to see if the patient begins to respond appropriately.

15. When an EMT-Intermediate deviates from the accepted standard of care that is recognized by law, it is known as:
    A. duty to act.
    B. proximate cause.
    C. negligence.
    D. breach of duty.

16. An EMT-Intermediate fails to properly check and maintain his EMS equipment. In a negligence suit, his action may be considered as:
    A. failure of duty to act.
    B. assault.
    C. abandonment.
    D. proximate cause.

17. Four elements must be demonstrated in a successful medical liability or negligent action case. These four elements are:
    A. duty, damages, battery, and proximate cause.
    B. consent, breach of duty, damages, and proximate cause.
    C. duty, breach of duty, damages, and proximate cause.
    D. consent, duty, damages, and proximate cause.

18. A legal obligation to provide care for a patient is known as:
    A. *res ipsa loquitur.*
    B. duty to act.
    C. consent.
    D. libel.

19. An EMT-Intermediate who touches a person without his or her consent may be charged with:
    A. battery.
    B. assault.
    C. slander.
    D. abandonment.

20. Turning the care and management of a critical patient over to a health care provider without ensuring that a greater or equal level of care will be provided is called:
    A. *res ipsa loquitur.*
    B. abandonment.
    C. libel.
    D. slander.

21. Injuring a person's character in writing is called:
    A. slander.
    B. assault.
    C. battery.
    D. libel.

22. Which of the following statements is an example of slander?
    A. Male patient states he "snorted coke all day."
    B. We are en route with a 70-year-old female in cardiac arrest.
    C. Patient was ejected from the vehicle during a high-speed chase.
    D. The drunk was found in a field under his car.

23. Which of the following patients could receive emergency care on the basis of implied consent?
    A. 10-year-old male pedestrian hit by a car while on a school field trip.
    B. 82-year-old female found unconscious in a restaurant.
    C. 16-year-old female driver of a car involved in a low speed collision.
    D. 3-year-old male with a minor laceration after falling at day care.

24. Many states require notification of the appropriate authorities when health care workers suspect child abuse or abuse of the elderly, evidence of violent crimes, and:

A. accidents involving motor vehicles.

B. patients who have ingested illegal drugs.

C. emergencies that threaten the public health.

D. potential medical malpractice.

25. You are washing the ambulance in front of the station when a frantic child runs up to you and says that his mom cut her hand real bad. After he gives you his address, you tell him you'll be right there after you get your partner. Given this situation, which of the following best describes your duty to act?

A. You have no duty to act since the child is a minor.

B. You have a duty to act since you told the child you would be right there.

C. You have no duty to act since dispatch did not use the alert tones.

D. You have a duty to act because you were at the station.

26. You have a competent patient who refuses to go with you to the hospital. A police officer on scene will not place him under protective custody, but orders you to transport. Which of the following best describes your actions if you transport the patient?

A. You may be held liable for false imprisonment.

B. You may be held liable for slander.

C. You may be held liable for a criminal case.

D. The police have the authority to dictate care and transport of patients.

27. Which one of the following types of consent will provide the best defense from a charge of battery?

A. implied consent

B. informed consent

C. expressed consent

D. assumed consent

28. The lawsuit against an EMT-Intermediate as a result of performing improper spinal immobilization on a patient is based on:

A. criminal law.

B. tort law.

C. battery.

D. assault.

29. An EMT-Intermediate is interviewed by the news media following a call to an elected official's home. He states that the patient is a drug addict and was found in the bathroom suffering from an overdose. The EMT-I can be charged with which of the following?

A. libel

B. negligence

C. assault

D. slander

30. An EMT-Intermediate tells an intoxicated patient, "I am going to stick this big needle in your arm if you don't cooperate." This EMT-Intermediate could be charged with which of the following?

A. battery

B. libel

C. false imprisonment

D. assault

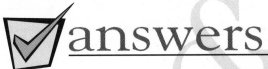

answers & rationales

1.

B. When a patient is made aware of the emergency medical care and risk and agrees, he or she has provided informed consent. Before a patient can provide informed consent the patient must understand: (1) the nature of the illness or injury, (2) the recommended treatment, (3) the possible or foreseeable risks and dangers that may result from the treatment, (4) possible alternative treatments and risks, and (5) the dangers of refusing treatment. *(1.3.2g)*

2.

D. In this case, advanced life support care was initiated; consequently, turning care over to a BLS unit would be abandonment. EMS personnel must remain with the patient until the patient is under the care of other EMS personnel of equal or greater training. *(1.3.2j)*

3.

A. Contact with medical control is irrelevant to the process of proving negligence. In order to prove negligence, four elements are required: (1) the EMT-Intermediate had a duty to perform, (2) the EMT-Intermediate breached their duty by not upholding the standard of care, (3) injury occurred to the patient, (4) the actions or inactions of the EMT-Intermediate caused the injury. *(1.3.5)*

4.

A. The child should be treated under the doctrine of implied consent. The EMT-Intermediate has the responsibility to treat the child because of the possi-

ble life threat. Neither child is old enough to sign a refusal. Attempts to contact the parents should be delegated to law enforcement at the scene or, by the emergency department staff. *(1.3.2i)*

5.

B. Threatening your patient with an unwanted procedure would fall under assault. Assault refers to placing someone in fear or apprehension of bodily harm. Performing the unwanted procedure could be battery (unlawful touching of a person). Libel is false or malicious writings and slander is false or malicious spoken words. *(1.3.2l)*

6.

C. Reasonable force may be used to restrain a violent patient. However, not all mental health laws allow patients to be transported and hospitalized against their will. EMT-Intermediates need to be familiar with their jurisdictions. Police authorization may not always be necessary, but it is a definite legal advantage. *(1.3.7)*

7.

A. Implied consent is used to provide emergency care for patients with altered mental states, or those who are unresponsive or who cannot make a rational decision. *(1.3.2h)*

8.

A. The writing of false or malicious statements defines an act of libel. As such, writing that a person is "a drunk" would be an example of a libelous act. Verbally saying that to the ED physician would be an example of slander. Writing or saying that the patient, "claims she was raped" is not an act of slander or liable. For in the latter instance, the EMT-Intermediate is merely reporting what the patient specifically said. *(1.3.2k)*

Good Samaritan Laws, protect people from liability for assisting at the scene of a medical emergency. Delegation of Authority means that EMT-Intermediates may only practice under the auspices of a licensed physician. *(1.3.1)*

9.

C. If the EMT-Intermediate fails to obtain proper consent from the patient prior to initiating care, he or she may be charged with battery. An abandonment charge would stem from leaving the patient in the care of a lesser trained individual, or by leaving the patient without care. Slander is damaging a person's character by false or malicious words. *(1.3.6)*

14.

A. You can proceed with treatment of this patient under implied consent. Implied consent is used when the patient has an altered mental status and it is assumed, or implied, that the patient would want to be treated. *(1.3.2i)*

10.

D. Applying the nasal cannula without the patient's consent amounts to battery. Even though your protocol states oxygen should be administered, consent must always be obtained. *(1.3.2e)*

15.

C. Negligence is a deviation from the standard of care. Duty to act, proximate cause, breach of duty, and injury must be proven in order to be held negligent. *(1.3.2a)*

11.

D. You have received expressed consent. Expressed consent grants you the right to treat the patient and can occur in writing, verbally, or by gestures. In this instance, the expressed consent consisted of a nod and a moan. The consent is not informed because the risks and benefits of the intervention were not fully explained. Also, the consent is not implied because the patient did respond with acknowledgement. *(1.3.2h)*

16.

D. Failure to provide care and check and maintain equipment to an acceptable standard of care is sufficient grounds for a negligence action. You are expected to provide EMS care at the same level a "prudent" EMT-Intermediate would provide under the same or similar circumstances. A "prudent" EMT-Intermediate would maintain equipment and supplies in a high state of readiness. Failure of equipment may be a proximate cause of death or injury. *(1.3.2a)*

12.

A. The fact that the patient self-extricated himself from the vehicle is of prime importance in documentation. If this patient has a spinal injury that has been worsened by his independent actions, documentation must reflect this so as you are not held responsible for the worsening of this patient's condition. *(1.3.3)*

17.

C. Four items must be demonstrated in a case of negligence in order for the action to be successful. The four items are: duty to perform (a legal obligation to provide care for the patient, also referred to as a duty to act), breach of duty (inappropriate standard of care), damages (the patient was injured by the breach of duty), and proximate cause (there is a direct relationship between the damages sustained and the breach of duty). *(1.3.2b)*

13.

D. The State Medical Practice Act defines the scope and role of the EMT-Intermediate on the state level.

18.

B. An obligation to provide care for a patient is known as duty to act. It may be a contractual obligation similar to a contract between a governmental agency and a private provider of EMS. The duty to act is clear in areas serviced by government-provided EMS services. The governmental agency has a "duty to respond or act" to provide care and assistance to the citizen's served. *(1.3.2d)*

19.

A. Battery occurs with the unlawful touching of another person without that person's consent. Assault requires the person to be in immediate fear of bodily harm with or without touching. Slander is the act of injuring a person's character by false, spoken words. Abandonment occurs when care is ended without a transfer of care to an appropriately trained individual. *(1.3.2e)*

20.

B. Abandonment can occur in one of two common situations; when initiating and then discontinuing care without transfer, or by releasing a patient to a lesser level of care. *(1.3.2j)*

21.

D. Harming a person's character, name, or reputation by writing is called libel. The use of words or making false verbal statements is called slander. Battery is touching without consent. Assault is an action that places a person in fear of bodily harm. *(1.3.2k)*

22.

D. Slander is the act of injuring a person's character or reputation by malicious spoken words. When providing patient information over the radio or to other health care professionals, the EMT-Intermediate should limit oral communication to essential and non-judgmental matters of patient care. It would not be appropriate to make a statement such as, "The drunk was found in a field under his car." However, if the patient admits he "snorted coke all day" it is appropriate to report. *(1.3.2f)*

23.

B. Implied consent is used in situations involving a patient who is unconscious and/or unresponsive. Care is initiated under the premise that the patient would desire care if they were conscious and able to make the decision. *(1.3.2i)*

24.

C. Many states require notification of the appropriate authorities when health care workers suspect child abuse or abuse of the elderly, evidence of violent crimes, and emergencies that threaten the public health such as dog bites. *(1.3.4)*

25.

B. Duty to act is evoked as soon as the EMS agency states that help is on the way, regardless of who summoned the ambulance in the first place, or how the call was dispatched. So the fact that the child was a minor, or the patient is an adult is not relevant. Because you are at the station does not mean you have a duty to act, for example, your unit could be out of service for decontamination procedures. *(1.3.2d)*

26.

A. If a police officer requests you to transport a competent patient, but is unwilling to take responsibility by placing the patient under protective custody, you cannot transport that patient unless you have the patient's consent. Even if you provide just transport without treatment, you can be held liable for false imprisonment. *(1.3.2m)*

27.

B. Of the types of consent listed, informed consent is the strongest because not only is the person agreeing to let you care for him or her (expressed consent), the person fully understands what it is you're going to do to him or her during the treatment phase. *(1.3.2g)*

28.

B. Tort law is a branch of civil law that deals with civil actions committed by one person against another. Malpractice litigation is handled under tort law. *(1.3.2c)*

29.

D. Injuring a person's character, name, or reputation by false and malicious spoken words is slander. To accuse a person openly in public of being a drug addict would be an example of slander. *(1.3.2f)*

30.

D. Threatening a patient with a large needle would be considered assault. Assault is creating apprehension of immediate bodily harm without consent. *(1.3.2l)*

4 Medical Terminology

chapter objectives

Questions in this chapter relate to DOT objectives 1.4.1–1.4.6. Please see the Appendix for more information.

DIRECTIONS Each of the questions or incomplete statements below is followed by suggested answers or completions. Select the **one answer** that is best in each case.

---

1. You are treating a patient who has a history of hepatitis. This patient is suffering from:
   A. disease of the hepatic duct.
   B. inflammation of the liver.
   C. disease of the kidneys.
   D. inflammation of the kidneys.

2. In reference to the lower extremity, the knee lies _____ to the ankle.
   A. medial
   B. lateral
   C. proximal
   D. distal

3. You are transporting a patient from a nursing home to the hospital. The patient's chart indicates that this patient has a history of RHD. RHD is the medical abbreviation for:
   A. rheumatic heart disease.
   B. right heart disease.
   C. right hand deficit.
   D. regular history of diabetes.

4. You are on-line with the medical control physician. She asks if the patient presents with circumoral cyanosis. She wants to know if the patient has:
   A. bluish color to the fingernail beds.
   B. difficulty speaking.
   C. swelling of the face.
   D. blueness around the mouth.

5. You are dispatched to a local nursing home for an elderly patient who is having difficulty speaking. You would document this as:
   A. dysphagia.
   B. dyspnea.
   C. dysphasia.
   D. polyphagia.

6. You are treating a patient who has a history of urinary bladder inflammation. Which medical term pertains to this patient's history?
   A. cholecystitis
   B. cystitis
   C. otitis
   D. phlebitis

7. You are transporting a patient to the emergency department for difficulty breathing. While obtaining the patient's medical history you find he or she is taking a well-known antibiotic t.i.d. The abbreviation t.i.d. means:
   A. four times a day.
   B. three times a day.
   C. takes as needed.
   D. two times a day.

8. While transporting a 43-year-old female patient she informs you she is being treated for nephritis. You associate this term with which organ?
   A. the liver
   B. the kidneys
   C. the stomach
   D. the intestines

9. You are treating a gentleman who started having problems breathing after he went to bed for the evening. He only has problems breathing when laying flat. What term best describes this patient's complaint?
   A. hypopnea
   B. cyanosis
   C. hypoxia
   D. orthopnea

10. The use of appropriate medical terminology would **not** be appropriate when communicating with:

    A. the patient.
    B. the patient's sister who is a nurse.
    C. the ED physician.
    D. the medical dispatcher.

11. Which of the following statements is correct regarding the position of the trachea to other thoracic structures?

    A. The trachea is posterior to the esophagus.
    B. The trachea is lateral to the carina.
    C. The trachea is inferior to the diaphragm.
    D. The trachea is medial to the lungs.

12. While reviewing a prehospital care report, you encounter the abbreviation "gtt." This refers to:

    A. Glasgow trauma total.
    B. milliliter.
    C. drop.
    D. none of the above.

13. While assessing a male patient with diffuse abdominal pain, he tells you he was recently diagnosed with "cholecystitis." You identify this as an inflammation of the:

    A. gall bladder.
    B. spleen.
    C. kidney.
    D. nerves.

14. Which of the following suffixes refers to weakness?

    A. -plegia
    B. -paresis
    C. -phagia
    D. -pathy

15. While assessing a patient involved in a diving accident you note an absence of motor function on the right side and extreme weakness on the left. Which of the following statements represents the most appropriate documentation of this condition?

    A. right hemiplegia and left hemiparesis
    B. left hemiplegia and right-sided weakness
    C. right quadriplegia and left-sided paresis
    D. left quadriplegia and right-sided paresis

16. While assessing a 72-year-old female patient who fell, you note that her left leg seems rotated outward. When communicating with on-line medical control how would you correctly describe the left lower extremity?

    A. flexed
    B. laterally rotated
    C. adducted
    D. medially rotated

17. At a nursing home, a staff RN informs you that your patient's chief complaint is hyperpyrexia and was just given 750 mg of Tylenol p.o. You recognize this as:

    A. Tylenol by mouth.
    B. Tylenol per order of physician.
    C. Tylenol by suppository.
    D. Tylenol followed by water.

18. A 76-year-old female suffers from dysphagia. This pertains to:

    A. without speech.
    B. without eating.
    C. difficulty swallowing.
    D. difficulty speaking.

19. Your adult patient is breathing 40 times a minute. This is known as:

    A. tachycardia.
    B. bradycardia.
    C. tachypnea.
    D. bradypnea.

20. While assessing your patient she states she had an oophorectomy last month. You know this to be:
    A. visual examination of the airway.
    B. inflammation of the vocal cords.
    C. surgical removal of cataracts.
    D. surgical excision of the ovary.

21. Your patient states he is experiencing pain when he urinates. The medical term is:
    A. dysuria.
    B. polyuria.
    C. hematuria.
    D. lipoiduria.

22. Your patient has a GSW below the shoulder blade. You document this on your medical report as:
    A. intercostal.
    B. supraclavicular.
    C. infrascapular.
    D. intralobar.

23. Your patient's pupils are equal and reactive to light. Which of these is an acceptable medical abbreviation?
    A. Pupils E/R
    B. Pupils ERL
    C. PERL
    D. PEARTL

24. The nurse is giving you report on a patient you will be transporting. He states the patient is medicated q.i.d. How often does the patient receive medication?
    A. once a day
    B. twice a day
    C. three times a day
    D. four times a day

25. Which of the following root words describes a muscle that closes an opening when it contracts?
    A. sphincter
    B. asthenia
    C. glomerulus
    D. cochlea

26. Which of the following prefixes refers to the blood vessels?
    A. cerebro-
    B. hemato-
    C. pulmo-
    D. angio-

27. Macro- is to micro- as hyper- is to:
    A. hyster-.
    B. dys-.
    C. orchi-.
    D. hypo-.

28. Supine is to prone as medial is to:
    A. lateral.
    B. ventral.
    C. dorsal.
    D. superior.

29. A fracture at the upper end of the upper arm bone would be described as:
    A. a proximal tibial fracture.
    B. a distal tibial fracture.
    C. a distal humerus fracture.
    D. a proximal humerus fracture.

30. An imaginary vertical line that separates the anterior lateral chest from the posterior lateral chest is called the:
    A. anterior axillary line.
    B. mid-axillary line.
    C. scapular line.
    D. posterior axillary line.

31. Which medical abbreviation is incorrectly defined?
    A. GI—gastrointestinal
    B. Dx—dyspnea
    C. cc—cubic centimeter
    D. c/o—complains of

32. Which medical abbreviation is incorrectly defined?
    A. L—liter
    B. RBC—red blood cell
    C. WNL—within normal limits
    D. q—drop

33. Which root word is incorrectly defined?
    A. stern—chest
    B. pod—back
    C. rhin—nose
    D. xen—foreign

34. Which prefix is incorrectly defined?
    A. cephal—large
    B. neo—new
    C. epi—upon
    D. auto—self

35. Which of the following terms are opposites?
    A. anterior—ventral
    B. lateral—medial
    C. posterior—dorsal
    D. superior—cranial

36. A patient who is complaining of shortness of breath is said to have:
    A. dyspnea.
    B. dystachea.
    C. apnea.
    D. tachypnea.

37. The portion of the humerus that is closest to the shoulder is the:
    A. distal end of the humerus.
    B. medial end of the humerus.
    C. inferior end of the humerus.
    D. proximal end of the humerus.

38. Your partner tells you that the patient has a large open laceration to the occipital portion of her head. The laceration is located on the:
    A. top of the head.
    B. side of the head.
    C. back of the head.
    D. front of the head.

39. Dispatch informs you that you have a patient with hematemesis. You know this as:
    A. coughing up blood.
    B. urinating blood.
    C. vomiting blood.
    D. blood in the stool.

40. Which of the following prefixes refers to the head:
    A. cerebr-
    B. cephal-
    C. cyan-
    D. cerv-

41. You are reviewing a run sheet in which the EMT-I used the abbreviation "CHF." You know this means:
    A. chronic heart flutter.
    B. chronic hepatic failure.
    C. congestive heart failure.
    D. calcified humoral fracture.

42. In describing the location of a laceration which is located between the elbow and wrist, which of the following is most correct?
    A. The laceration is proximal to the elbow.
    B. The laceration is lateral to the pelvis.
    C. The laceration is distal to the elbow.
    D. The laceration is medial to the wrist.

43. Which of the following terms means an abnormally slow heart rate?
    A. bradycardia
    B. bradycephalia
    C. bradypnea
    D. bradykinin

44. Which of the following terms are opposites?
    A. hypopnea—hypoventilation
    B. medial—midline
    C. superior—cephalad
    D. proximal—distal

45. You want to use an abbreviation on your run sheet which represents someone who has difficulty breathing with any physical activity. This abbreviation would be:
    A. DOA.
    B. DOE.
    C. MAE.
    D. Dx.

46. You are transferring a patient from the emergency department to another hospital. The physician tells you the patient is NPO. This means the patient:
    A. cannot receive oxygen by mask.
    B. is allergic to nitroglycerin.
    C. should not be resuscitated.
    D. cannot have anything by mouth.

47. You are assessing a patient who states he has had hemiparesis for the last few days. He is complaining of which of the following?
    A. paralysis to his lower legs
    B. weakness to one side of his body
    C. tingling to one side of his body
    D. weakness to the lower part of his body

48. Which of the following medical terms would describe a patient who complains of very frequent and excessive urination?
    A. oliguria
    B. hematuria
    C. polyuria
    D. dysuria

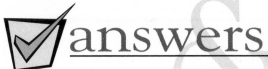
answers & rationales

1.

B. This patient has an inflammation of the liver. The prefix *hepat-* means liver and the suffix *-itis* means inflammation. *(1.4.1)*

2.

C. The knee is closer to the heart than the ankle. This would make it proximal. *(1.4.2)*

3.

A. The medical abbreviation RHD stands for rheumatic heart disease. *(1.4.3)*

4.

D. Circumoral cyanosis means "a blue discoloration around the mouth." *(1.4.5)*

5.

C. The patient is suffering from dysphasia. The prefix *dys-* means difficulty and the suffix *-phasia* means speech. The suffix *-phagia* means eating, and *-pnea* means breathing. *(1.4.1)*

6.

B. An inflammation of the urinary bladder is cystitis. The prefix *cyst-* means bladder and the suffix *-itis* means inflammation. The prefix *cholecyst-* means gall bladder, *ot-* refers to the ear, and *phleb-* is a vein. *(1.4.2)*

7.

B. The abbreviation t.i.d. means three times a day. A medication taken two times a day is abbreviated b.i.d., and four times a day is q.i.d. PRN means as needed. *(1.4.3)*

8.

B. *Nephr-* refers to the kidney, *enter-* refers to the intestines, *gastr-* refers to the stomach, and *hepat-* refers to the liver. *(1.4.4)*

9.

D. Orthopnea is the best term for documentation because it refers to being unable to breathe while laying flat. Cyanosis and hypoxia may result from the scenario but are not adequate terms to describe this patient. Hypopnea is inadequate ventilatory volume. *(1.4.5)*

10.

A. It would be best to talk to the patient in words he or she can understand. Rarely will patients have a good grasp on medical terminology, so they should receive information in a way that they can understand. Medical terminology should be used when conversing with other people involved in caring for a patient both outside and inside the hospital. The use of medical terminology ensures better communication, and it lessens the opportunity for statements to be ambiguous. *(1.4.1)*

11.

D. The location of the trachea can be defined by its medial positioning between each lung. Integral to properly communicating data to the emergency staff is the ability to describe anatomical injuries or landmarks appropriately. This ability will only come from the working knowledge of anatomical terms used in emergency medicine. All other descriptions for the position of the trachea are incorrect. *(1.4.2)*

12.

C. The abbreviation "gtt" refers to "drop." Having a thorough understanding of common medical abbreviations will allow you to prepare a more concise written report quickly. However, using the abbreviations appropriately is a must. *(1.4.3)*

13.

A. Cholecystitis refers to an inflammation of the gall bladder. *Cholecyst-* means gall bladder, and *-itis* means inflammation. Root words are the portion of the medical term which define the basic meaning of the word. The root words can then be modified by prefixes and suffixes. *(1.4.4)*

14.

B. The suffix *-paresis* refers to weakness. You may see the same suffix on the end of various root words. For example, paraparesis and hemiparesis refer to weakness of the legs or one half of the body respectively. The suffix *-phagia* refers to swallowing and *-pathy* refers to disease. *(1.4.5)*

15.

A. This patient presents with right hemiplegia (half paralysis) and left hemiparesis (half weakness). The prefix *quad-* refers to all four extremities. *(1.4.1)*

16.

B. The patient's left leg is laterally rotated or turned away from the midline of the body. *(1.4.2)*

17.

A. The abbreviation p.o. refers to anything given by mouth. None of the other options represent this definition. *(1.4.3)*

18.

C. The patient has dysphagia. The prefix *dys-* translates to difficulty while *-phagia* refers to eating or swallowing. *(1.4.5)*

19.

C. The patient's condition is called tachypnea, *tachy-* is the prefix for fast and *-pnea* is the common root word for breathing. *Brady-* is the prefix for slow and *-cardia* is the root word for heart, thus slow heart rate. *(1.4.1a)*

20.

D. An oophorectomy is the surgical removal of the ovary. *Oophor-* is the prefix for ovary and *-ectomy* is the suffix meaning to cut out or excise. *(1.4.1b)*

21.

A. Painful urination is dysuria. *Dys-* is with pain or difficulty and *-uria* has to do with urine. Polyuria is many or frequent urination. Hematuria is blood in the urine. Lipoiduria is lipids or fats in the urine. *(1.4.2a)*

22.

C. Document the GSW (gunshot wound) as being infrascapular. *Infra-* is below and *-scapular* is scapula or shoulder blade. Intercostal is between the ribs. Supraclavicular is above the clavicle. Intralobar is within a lobe. *(1.4.2b)*

23.

C. The correct medical abbreviation for pupils that are equal and reactive to light is PERL. *(1.4.3a)*

24.

D. The abbreviation q.i.d. is four times a day. Twice a day is b.i.d., and three times a day is t.i.d. *(1.4.3b)*

25.

A. Sphincter describes a muscle that closes an opening when it contracts. This type of muscle can be found in the bladder, stomach, and rectum. *(1.4.4)*

26.

D. *Angio-* refers to the blood vessels. An example of this is angioplasty, which is repairing a blood vessel. *Cerebro-* refers to the brain, *hemato-* refers to the blood. *Pulmo-* refers to the lungs. *(1.4.5)*

27.

D. *Macro-* is a prefix that means large, and *micro-* is a prefix that means small. *Hyper-* means over or excessive, and *hypo-* means under or deficient. *Dys-* translates as with difficulty, *orchi-* is testicle, and *hyster-* pertains to the uterus. *(1.4.1)*

28.

A. Supine is lying face up, while prone is laying face down. Medial is toward the midline, and lateral is away from the midline. Ventral is toward the front, and dorsal is toward the back. Superior is toward the top. *(1.4.1)*

29.

D. The humerus is the upper arm bone, and proximal means closer to the top or origin, so this injury would best be described as a proximal humoral fracture. The tibia is the anterior bone of the lower leg, and distal means away from the point of attachment. *(1.4.2)*

30.

B. The mid-axillary line separates the anterior chest from the posterior chest. This is a vertical line located at the midline of the axilla or the armpit. *(1.4.2)*

31.

B. Dx is the abbreviation for diagnosis. *(1.4.3)*

32.

D. *q-* means every. The abbreviation for drop is gtt. *(1.4.3)*

33.

B. *Pod-* refers to foot. *(1.4.4)*

34.

A. *Cephal-* refers to the head. The suffix *-megaly* refers to large. *(1.4.5)*

35.

B. Lateral and medial are the opposite terms. Lateral means away from the midline of the body, while medial means toward the midline of the body. *(1.4.1)*

36.

A. The term dyspnea refers to shortness of breath. The prefix *dys-* means difficulty and *-pnea* is the common root word for breathing. *(1.4.1)*

37.

D. The part of the humerus that is closest to the shoulder is the proximal end. Proximal is the term that refers to being closest to the heart while distal is furthest from the heart. The distal end of the humerus is near the elbow. *(1.4.2)*

38.

C. The occipital area of the skull is at the back of the head. The frontal refers to the front (forehead), temporal is the side, and parietal is the top. *(1.4.2)*

39.

C. Hematemisis is defined as vomiting up blood, while hemoptysis is defined as coughing up blood. Blood found in the urine is called hematuria. *(1.4.1)*

40.

B. The prefix referring to the head is *cephal-*. *Cerebr-* generally refers to the brain. *Cerv-* refers to the cervical region of the spinal column and *cyan-* means bluish color. *(1.4.3)*

41.

C. CHF stands for the medical condition known as congestive heart failure. All of the other answers are fictitious names using the abbreviation CHF. *(1.4.2)*

42.

C. A laceration between the elbow and wrist could be phrased as a laceration occurring distal to the elbow. In describing injury locations, the EMT-I needs to know appropriate terminology to describe locations. Distal means away from the heart and proximal means closer to the heart. Lateral means to the sides and medial means towards the midline. *(1.4.5)*

43.

A. Bradycardia is an abnormally slow heart rate, *brady-* means slow, and *-cardia* is the root word for heart. Bradypnea refers to an abnormally slow respiratory rate, *-pnea* is the root word for breathing. *(1.4.1)*

44.

D. Proximal and distal are opposite terms and are used for referencing locations on the body. Hypopnea and hypoventilation refer to abnormally shallow breathing. Medial means towards the midline. Finally, superior means a position above another, and cephalad means towards the head. *(1.4.4)*

45.

B. DOE stands for dyspnea on exertion. This is the abbreviation that should be used for a patient who is having difficulty breathing with any physical activity. *(1.4.3)*

46.

D. The medical abbreviation NPO means nothing by mouth. *(1.4.3)*

47.

B. The patient has weakness to one side of his body. The prefix *hemi-* refers to half of the body if split into a right and left side; *-paresis* means weakness. *(1.4.4)*

48.

C. A patient with polyuria is suffering from frequent and excessive urination. *Poly-* means many or excessive, and *-uria* refers to urine. *(1.4.4)*

5 EMS Communications

chapter objectives

Questions in this chapter relate to DOT objectives 1.5.1–1.5.21. Please see the Appendix for more information.

DIRECTIONS Each of the questions or incomplete statements below is followed by suggested answers or completions. Select the **one answer** that is best in each case.

1. Responsibilities of the emergency medical dispatcher include all of the following, **except**:
   A. acting as the initial contact with the public.
   B. allocating the appropriate resources for the emergency response.
   C. diagnosing the medical problem of the patient.
   D. alerting EMS personnel and directing them to the scene.

2. In order to ensure that radio transmission is clear, all of the following guidelines should be followed, **except**:
   A. press the transmit button for 1 second before speaking.
   B. speak slowly and clearly into or across a microphone that is at close range.
   C. speak in a normal pitch and know what information you are going to relay before transmitting.
   D. communicate to the hospital using codes when possible.

3. When utilizing a portable radio transmitter/receiver, which position of the antenna will provide the maximum transmitting range?
   A. pointed horizontal and low
   B. pointed vertical and as high as possible
   C. pointed horizontal and high
   D. perpendicular to any large metal object

4. A major limitation of the 10-code system is:
   A. codes shorten air transmission time.
   B. codes enable transmission of clear and concise information.

C. medical information is often too complex to code.
D. codes promote patient confidentiality.

5. During a medical emergency you decide to initiate an IV of normal saline during transport of the patient to a local facility. All of your actions are authorized by:
   A. American Medical Association guidelines.
   B. US-DOT curriculum objectives.
   C. protocols.
   D. on-line medical control.

6. The batteries of a portable radio should be replaced:
   A. after each call.
   B. after the current battery is dead.
   C. at the beginning of each new shift.
   D. on a daily basis.

7. Of the following, which is the **least** important for the EMS dispatcher to get at the time of the call?
   A. the location of the call.
   B. the closest cross-street to the call.
   C. the callback number.
   D. the nature of the call.

8. While giving your radio report to the receiving hospital, the ED physician gives you a treatment order which you believe to be absolutely inappropriate for your patient. You should:
   A. perform the order exactly as directed to.
   B. tell the physician you refuse to do that.
   C. acknowledge the orders, but do not perform them.
   D. repeat the orders, exactly as given, back to the ED physician.

9. A typical EMS event is said to consist of several components. These can include: event detection and notification of EMS, response of EMS, treatment, transport, and delivery to the hospital. All of these components are linked by:
   A. medical control.
   B. medical protocols.
   C. medical personnel.
   D. communications.

10. While in the living room of a house, you experience difficulty contacting dispatch on your portable radio. What corrective action can be taken to improve the transmitting ability of your radio?
    A. adjust the squelch
    B. stand up when transmitting
    C. pause 2 to 3 seconds before speaking into the microphone
    D. point the antenna towards an open window or door

11. At a minimum, which one of the following must be attained by the EMS call-taker prior to dispatching the ambulance?
    A. phone number from which the caller is calling
    B. existing hazards on the scene
    C. patient's level of consciousness
    D. age of the patient

12. Identify the radio equipment that can receive a transmission from a low-power source on one frequency, and then re-transmit it at a higher power on another frequency.
    A. telemetry
    B. repeater
    C. encoder
    D. modulator

13. To improve the life expectancy of radio equipment, you should clean them using:

    A. water and a cleaning solvent.
    B. cloth dampened with toluene.
    C. damp cloth and mild detergent.
    D. copious amounts of hot water.

14. All of the following are proper radio transmission techniques, **except**:
    A. use codes whenever possible.
    B. press the button for 1 second before talking.
    C. speak slowly and clearly, avoid difficult words.
    D. use the "echo" system when receiving directions.

15. You are unable to contact medical control online; you should:
    A. contact dispatch for medical direction.
    B. refer to your standing orders.
    C. provide no additional medical treatment.
    D. immediately call for another EMS unit.

16. All of the following are acceptable and pertinent information to relay to a receiving hospital by radio, **except**:
    A. patient's name.
    B. patient's age.
    C. patient's complaint.
    D. patient's weight.

17. Of the following sequences which is the most organized way to communicate information to a physician?
    A. description of scene, patient's age, chief complaint, physical exam, treatment given
    B. patient's age, description of the scene, chief complaint, physical exam, treatment given
    C. chief complaint, description of the scene, patient's age, physical exam, treatment given
    D. physical exam, patient's age, description of the scene, chief complaint, treatment given

18. The **first** link in the EMS communication chain is:
    A. communication between the EMT-Intermediate and medical control.
    B. completion of a written report.
    C. dispatch of EMS unit.
    D. notification of EMS dispatch.

19. The position of the antenna on a portable transmitter/receiver radio should be positioned _____ to provide maximum coverage of the transmitted signal.
    A. obliquely
    B. horizontally
    C. vertically
    D. laterally

20. One advantage of a repeater radio system over a nonrepeater system is:
    A. the handheld portables used with a repeater system will typically have a higher watt output.
    B. the repeater system does not have to use "voting."
    C. in large geographic areas, it reduces simultaneous transmitting of two portable radios.
    D. There is no advantage to the use of a repeater system over a nonrepeater system.

21. One of the major purposes for providing a radio report of patient information to hospital personnel while en route is to:
    A. provide a description of treatments provided.
    B. allow the hospital to begin preparations for patient arrival.
    C. provide a chief complaint of the patient's condition.
    D. provide a Trauma Index or Glasgow Coma Score.

22. Which of the following does **not** need to be included in your radio report to hospital personnel?
    A. unit name and number of patients
    B. patient's age, sex, and weight
    C. patient's complete medical history
    D. patient's chief complaint

23. All of the following statements about the written EMS run report are true, **except**:
    A. the documentation allows for personal opinions about the patient.
    B. it provides a record of the patient's initial condition and care.
    C. it documents a patient's refusal of care and transport.
    D. it becomes a legal record of the prehospital care.

24. What is the function of a remote console in an EMS communications system?
    A. It limits the amount of wear and tear on the base station.
    B. It can be used to retransmit signals from a lower frequency.
    C. It allows complete operation of the base station from any location.
    D. It enables portable radios to have telemetry capability.

25. The Federal Communications Commission controls and regulates radio communications through the allocation of frequencies and:
    A. establishing technical standards for radio equipment.
    B. licensing every EMS provider who communicates by radio.
    C. reviewing patient care reports for completeness and accuracy.
    D. conducting training programs for radio repair personnel.

26. Which one of the following responsibilities related to prehospital radio use does **not** belong to the Federal Communications Commission:
    A. assigns radio frequencies
    B. requires the use of special codes for EMS communication
    C. monitors frequencies for appropriate use
    D. grants site licenses for EMS base station transmitters

27. During a radio report to the hospital, you tell the receiving physician that you have defibrillated the patient at 200 joules and 300 joules. This information is useful to him for:
    A. proper billing purposes.
    B. to ensure that the patient is receiving optimal care.
    C. to allow him or her the opportunity to adequately prepare for your arrival.
    D. all of the above.

28. Which of the following are **not** routine aspects of daily radio maintenance for portable radios?
    A. ensuring the batteries are charged
    B. placing the radio in the leather case
    C. checking the radio for cracks
    D. programming in the pertinent radio frequencies

29. Of the following, which is the most appropriate order to relay patient information to the hospital?
    A. age, gender, vitals, chief complaint, assessment findings, past medical history
    B. chief complaint, vitals, age, transporting unit name and number
    C. gender, patient's physician, past medical history, vitals, assessment findings
    D. age, gender, chief complaint, medical history, vitals, assessment findings

30. Which of the following is **not** an example of one of the phases of communication in an EMS event?
    A. You contact your back-up crew to advise them of the situation and what equipment to bring into the scene.
    B. The crew is paged and notified of the nature and location of the call.
    C. The dispatcher contacts the police to respond to the scene.
    D. The EMT-I at the scene notifies the family of the patient of the seriousness of the illness.

31. Which of the following communication devices is responsible for receiving a transmission, boosting the power and then retransmitting it on another frequency?
    A. encoder
    B. repeater
    C. decoder
    D. remote console

32. The first person who can assist the patient begins with the:
    A. EMT-Paramedic.
    B. First Responder.
    C. Emergency Medical Dispatcher.
    D. EMT-Intermediate.

33. Which of the following techniques should be used to ensure proper and clear radio transmission?
    A. Hold the microphone 2 inches from your mouth and speak directly into it.
    B. Increase the pitch and volume of your voice when speaking.
    C. Use only codes to transmit information to avoid issues with patient confidentiality.
    D. Depress the push-to-talk button and wait 5 seconds before beginning your transmission.

34. The written EMS report following a call should:

   A. be discarded because of patient confidentiality issues.

   B. be filed with the hospital emergency department to ensure a continuum of care.

   C. not be used for billing purposes.

   D. not be used for collection of data because of the differences in patient care reporting among EMS personnel.

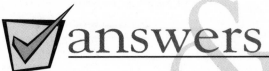

answers & rationales

1.

C. Although some EMS systems have the knowledge and capacity to provide medically approved pre-arrival instructions, the emergency medical dispatcher is not capable of diagnosing a patient's medical problem. Emergency medical dispatch is the nerve center of the EMS system. The emergency medical dispatcher is the initial, and perhaps the only contact with the public. The emergency medical dispatcher must be knowledgeable about all resources available in the system, and how to access them. *(1.5.7)*

2.

D. When communicating medical information to the hospital, codes can be confusing unless understood by everyone. Using plain English is the best way to reduce the likelihood of misinterpreted information. *(1.5.10)*

3.

B. Radio transmission ranges are maximized when the antenna is vertical and as high as possible. *(1.5.4)*

4.

C. One major limitation of radio codes is that medical information can be difficult to explain with a coding system. However, codes do shorten air time, are concise when understood, and provide patient confidentiality. *(1.5.9)*

5.

C. Starting an IV based on your own determination of the need is an action that is authorized by protocols, which are predetermined guidelines for prehospital care. On-line orders require contact with medical control. *(1.5.12)*

6.

D. Since the most common cause of radio malfunction is dead batteries they should be replaced on a daily basis. The intent of radio maintenance by the EMT-Intermediate is to ensure optimal radio performance. Replacing batteries too soon (for example, after each call or each shift) will decrease the battery's functional life due to multiple charging cycles. Waiting until the battery dies may leave you in a situation where you need it, but it will not work. *(1.5.3)*

7.

B. While all the mentioned bits of information are important, the cross streets for the call, while helpful, are not absolutely necessary. It is vital that the dispatcher have the location, nature, and callback number prior to dispatching the ambulance and any other necessary resources (police, fire, etc.). Ultimately, it is the EMT-Intermediate's responsibility to be familiar with the territory he/she responds to. *(1.5.8)*

8.

D. Since radio communications with the hospital may be difficult at times, you may receive an order that seems inappropriate. When this happens, utilize the "echo" technique, and repeat the orders back to the physician exactly as given for confirmation. This allows the physician the opportunity to review the orders and ensure that you heard them correctly. It is highly unlikely that the physician would direct you to do something "inappropriate." Irregular orders are usually the result of a misinformed physician or a communication failure. In either instance, echoing the orders back should clarify any discrepancies. *(1.5.11)*

9.

D. Communications play a vital role in linking the typical components of an EMS event. Medical control aids in the connection of transport and delivery, but does not apply to notification by the lay person. The same can be said of medical personnel, in that they are not required to link occurrence and actual detection. Finally, medical protocols are specific to patient care and cannot be said to link all of the components. *(1.5.1)*

10.

B. Standing up while transmitting often serves to improve transmitting ability. This action, in effect, raises the height of the antenna on the portable radio and increases coverage area. Adjusting the squelch and pausing before transmitting will not change transmitting ability. Since the antenna should remain as vertical as possible, pointing the antenna towards an open window or door would serve to decrease your ability for maximum transmission. *(1.5.4)*

11.

A. One of the items that must be attained by the EMS call-taker prior to dispatching the initial ambulance is the callback number so that they can be recontacted should they be disconnected. Other items that must be attained include the location and the nature of the event. The remaining answers provide information about the patient that is useful after the ambulance is already en route. *(1.5.8)*

12.

B. The repeater receives a transmission from a low-power portable or mobile radio and retransmits it on another frequency after boosting the power. Telemetry is the ability to transmit readings by radio. An encoder is a device for generating unique codes or tones that are recognized by decoders. A

modulator is a device that transforms electrical energy into sound waves. *(1.5.2)*

13.

C. Use only a water dampened cloth and a mild detergent. This will improve the appearance and performance. *(1.5.3)*

14.

A. Codes can be difficult to use in medical communications. If privacy is necessary, use the phone. Never use the patient's name over the radio. Pressing the button for one second before speaking will permit the repeater to function. Speaking slowly and clearly reduces confusion. By immediately repeating the directions, accurate confirmation will be accomplished. *(1.5.11)*

15.

B. If you cannot communicate with on-line medical direction, you should revert to "backup" written protocols or standing orders. Dispatch is not medical authority and will be of little assistance. You must provide appropriate and necessary treatment. Calling and waiting for an additional unit may delay treatment. *(1.5.12)*

16.

A. Transmitting the patient's name over the radio may cause a breach in patient confidentiality by permitting the name to be picked up on scanners and other radios. *(1.5.14)*

17.

A. After you introduce your unit call name or number and level of training, you should follow a systematic sequence like this one. One of the purposes of the radio report is to allow the hospital to prepare for your arrival. *(1.5.15)*

18.

D. This is the first of the five communication "phases" of a typical EMS event: 1) notification from the caller by 9-1-1 to EMS dispatch, 2) notification of appropriate EMS unit, 3) communications between EMT-Intermediate and medical control, 4) direct face-to-face communications with emergency department personnel, 5) notification of dispatch that the unit is back in service. *(1.5.1)*

19.

C. When using the portable radio, be sure to position the radio's antenna vertically to ensure maximum coverage during transmission and reception. *(1.5.4)*

20.

C. There are significant advantages to using a repeater system, especially in large geographic areas or areas with dense urban growth. The use of a repeater system prevents two portable radios from transmitting simultaneously because one portable cannot hear the other. Whether used in a repeater system or non-repeater system, the handheld portables all typically have a 1–5 watt, low power output. The repeater system requires the use of "voting" or determining which signal is the strongest then transmitting that signal. *(1.5.5)*

21.

B. There are two major purposes for radio communications with hospital personnel. The first is to allow the hospital staff time to prepare for treating the patient. The second is to obtain treatment orders from medical control. The other items that are listed are important to include in your report of the patient's condition, but not major reasons for verbal radio communications with hospital personnel. *(1.5.13)*

22.

C. While pertinent medical history is important, a complete medical history is not. Only those aspects of the patient's history that are relevant and pertinent should be included in your verbal radio report to the hospital. You want to "paint a picture" of the patient's condition to medical control. Including items that are irrelevant to the current problem may cause confusion. *(1.5.14)*

23.

A. The written EMS report is not the place to describe personal opinions of any kind. This includes disagreements related to treatments provided or not provided. Issues related to disagreements of a personal opinion should be expressed through an internal communication device such as an "Incident Report." *(1.5.16)*

24.

C. A remote console in an EMS communications system allows complete operation of the base station from any location by using dedicated telephone lines or microwave transmitter links. *(1.5.2)*

25.

A. The Federal Communications Commission (FCC) controls and regulates radio communications through allocating frequencies and establishing technical standards for radio equipment. *(1.5.6)*

26.

B. The FCC has numerous responsibilities regarding radio frequencies used by EMS personnel. They do not, however, require that a particular set of codes or signals be used. That decision is left up to the local EMS provider. *(1.5.6)*

27.

C. The primary reason the physician would want that information is so that he can prepare to assume treatment upon your arrival. That information may also be useful for assuring proper care delivery, but that is more of a role for the Quality Improvement Committee and not the physician directly. Billing comes after the trip is completed. *(1.5.13)*

28.

D. Rarely would the EMT-I have to keep programming the frequency numbers. These are often preset and cannot be altered by the field EMT-I. Portable radios take abuse in the prehospital environment and they should be inspected daily for cracks. To prevent further damage, they should also remain in the protective leather case as much as possible. And naturally, the EMT-I would want to assure the battery is fully charged prior to start of shift. *(1.5.3)*

29.

D. The radio report to the hospital needs to be relayed in a fashion that will allow hospital personnel to understand quickly the patient's current condition. This is a recommended format, while the first three responses are disorganized. *(1.5.15)*

30.

D. Notifying the family of the seriousness of the illness is not a link in EMS communication. Communication with dispatch, other crews, other public safety services, and the receiving hospital are all appropriate links in an EMS event. *(1.5.1)*

31.

B. A repeater receives a low-power transmission from a mobile or portable radio, boosts the power, and retransmits it on another frequency. *(1.5.2)*

32.

C. The emergency medical dispatcher is the first person to offer any type of emergency care for the patient prior to the arrival of any first responder or EMS unit. *(1.5.7)*

33.

A. The microphone should be held 2 to 3 inches from the mouth. Use a normal pitch and tone of voice to ensure clarity. Ten-codes are typically not used and have been replaced with the use of plain English. Once you have pressed the push-to-talk button, wait one second, then begin your transmission. *(1.5.10)*

34.

B. A copy of the EMS report must be filed with the hospital to ensure a proper continuum of care. The report is also used in billing and for other administrative reasons. The data collected from the EMS report is used in medical audits and is a major component in quality assurance and continuous quality improvement programs. *(1.5.16)*

6 General Patient Assessment and Initial Management

chapter objectives

Questions in this chapter relate to DOT objectives 1.6.1–1.6.67. Please see the Appendix for more information.

DIRECTIONS Each of the questions or incomplete statements below is followed by suggested answers or completions. Select the **one answer** that is best in each case.

1. Which of the following activities are done during the scene size-up?
   A. Determine mechanism of injury, identify, and treat immediate life threats.
   B. Gather information about present situation, question bystanders, and obtain past medical history.
   C. Complete physical exam, obtain baseline vital signs, and identify treatment priorities.
   D. Identify potential environmental or situational hazards, determine mechanism of injury, secure the scene, and locate patients.

2. You have responded to a call in which the patient was injured during a fight in the parking lot outside a bar. Although police are on scene a large hostile crowd gathers as you begin assessing the patient. What should you do to manage this situation?
   A. Leave the patient and return immediately to the ambulance.
   B. Use your body to shield the patient and continue your care.
   C. Move the patient to the ambulance with police assistance.
   D. Continue to provide care while the police deal with the crowd.

3. What is the primary difference in your approach to the assessment of a medical patient verses a trauma patient?
   A. Assessment of the trauma patient focuses on the relationship between the patient's past history and systemic physical findings.
   B. Assessment of the medical patient is directed toward signs of potential problems as suggested by the mechanism of injury.
   C. Assessment of the trauma patient tends to be more interactive with the patient based on detailed questioning of his or her past history.
   D. Assessment of the medical patient is more commonly directed toward gathering a history and performing a physical exam based on the reported symptoms.

4. The function of the vocal cords is to:
   A. regulate the passage of air into the trachea and control the production of sound.
   B. warm, filter, and humidify air as it enters the trachea thus decreasing the risk of bronchospasm.
   C. prevent aspiration because stimulation of the vocal cords triggers the gag reflex.
   D. secrete mucus, which traps particulate matter not filtered out in the upper airway.

5. Which of the following statements describes the flow of air from outside the body into the trachea?
   A. Air enters through the nose and mouth and moves through the vocal cords into the larynx, pharynx, and then into the trachea.
   B. Air enters through the oral pharynx and moves through the sinuses into the pharynx, through the larynx, and the trachea.
   C. Air enters the nose and then moves through the oral pharynx and through the larynx to the pharynx and into the trachea.

D. Air enters the nose and mouth and then moves into the pharynx where it enters the trachea via the larynx.

6. The function of turbinates in the nasopharynx is to:

A. warm and humidify air as it moves into the airway.

B. limit the amount of air that enters the airway.

C. divide the internal nasal cavity into two pathways of air entry.

D. serve as receptor sites to enhance the sense of smell.

7. Which of the following statements best describes the process of pulmonary ventilation?

A. Air moves into the lungs when the alveolar pressure exceeds the atmospheric pressure and moves out of the lungs when the alveolar pressure is less than the atmospheric pressure.

B. Air moves into the lungs when the pressure in the bronchi is greater than atmospheric pressure and moves out of the lungs when the bronchial pressure exceeds the atmospheric pressure.

C. Air moves into the lungs when the diaphragm relaxes, increasing the size of the thoracic cavity, and moves out of the lungs when the contraction of the diaphragm decreases the size of the thorax.

D. Air moves into the lungs when the alveolar pressure is lower than atmospheric pressure and moves out of the lungs when the alveolar pressure exceeds atmospheric pressure.

8. How is pulmonary ventilation affected by a diaphragmatic injury?

A. An injury to the diaphragm increases the potential size of the thoracic cavity and thus increases tidal volume with each respiration.

B. A diaphragmatic injury reduces oxygenation by limiting the amount of expansion of the uninjured lung caused by air in the pleural space.

C. An injury to the diaphragm impairs its ability to contract normally and reduces the potential size of the thoracic cavity during inhalation.

D. A diaphragmatic injury compromises ventilation when the accumulation of air in the pleural space and the resulting decrease in pressure maintain lung inflation.

9. An increase in airway resistance may be noticed when ventilating a patient due to all of the following, **except**:

A. tension pneumothorax.

B. occlusion of the airway.

C. esophageal intubation.

D. intubation of the right main stem bronchus.

10. A deflated reservoir bag observed while using a bag-valve-mask device may indicate all of the following, **except**:

A. an empty oxygen cylinder.

B. an increase in airway resistance.

C. a leak in the bag-valve-mask device.

D. a disconnected oxygen supply line.

11. Relative contraindications for oral tracheal intubation include an intact gag reflex, epiglottitis, and:

A. cardiac arrest.

B. cervical spine injury.

C. apnea secondary to an acute asthma attack.

D. hypoxic pulmonary edema patient in respiratory failure.

12. Which of the following statements regarding the use of a tourniquet for hemorrhage control is true?
    A. A sphygmomanometer is an effective tourniquet only if it is inflated to a minimum pressure of 300 mmHg.
    B. Inadequate tourniquet pressure will only inhibit venous return, thus increasing the rate and volume of blood loss.
    C. Tourniquets provide excellent control of hemorrhage and should be considered as first-line management in most situations.
    D. Once applied, tourniquets should be loosened after ten minutes to maintain perfusion of uninjured tissue adjacent to the wound.

13. Exposing the trauma patient during the rapid trauma assessment may result in:
    A. the development of life-threatening hypothermia.
    B. charges of assault and battery.
    C. quick identification of potentially life-threatening injuries.
    D. exacerbation of unstable cervical or thoracic spine injuries.

14. Of the following statements, which would be an important part of the pertinent past medical history for a 60-year-old male patient complaining of chest pain?
    A. Patient occassionally takes sinus medication.
    B. Patient had a hernia repair 2 years ago.
    C. Patient underwent coronary bypass surgery last year.
    D. Patient's brother died of a heart attack at the age of 78.

15. Which of the following activities would occur during the definitive care phase of the patient care continuum?

    A. administration of medications to control pain en route
    B. placement of a chest tube
    C. transmission of cardiac rhythms to the receiving facility
    D. ventilatory support via bag-valve-mask device

16. Which of the following statements most accurately describes the proper immobilization sequence for a supine patient?
    A. Manually stabilize the head and neck in a neutral position. Log roll the patient onto a long backboard. Strap the torso and legs securely to the board and then secure the patient's head and neck. Secure the backboard to the cot.
    B. Apply a cervical collar to stabilize the head and neck in a neutral position. Roll the patient onto a long backboard. Strap the patient securely to the board and secure the patient's head and neck. Secure the backboard to the cot.
    C. Manually stabilize the head and neck in a neutral position and apply a cervical collar. Log roll the patient onto a long backboard. Strap the torso and legs securely to the board and then secure the patient's head and neck. Secure the backboard to the cot.
    D. Apply a rigid collar to stabilize the head and neck in a neutral position. Log roll the patient onto the cot and strap the patient securely to prevent movement. Secure the patient's head and neck.

17. Which of the following activities should occur as part of your ongoing assessment of a patient while en route to the hospital?
    A. Report patient data to the receiving facility.

B. Reassess mental status, initial assessment, and vital signs every 5 or 15 minutes, and check interventions.

C. Reassure family members that the patient will be fine.

D. Document any care provided at the scene on the patient care report.

18. A 34-year-old male has collapsed in cardiac arrest as a result of choking on a cherry tomato. Two sets of abdominal thrusts and blind finger sweeps have failed to clear the obstruction. What would be your next action?

A. Continue abdominal thrusts and call for ALS and transport.

B. Begin cardiopulmonary resuscitation.

C. Suction the airway and begin ventilation.

D. Perform chest compressions only without ventilation.

19. A 73-year-old Alzheimer's patient is found sitting on the steps of a residence at 2:00 A.M. The patient is wet, disoriented, and has a decreased mental status. Which of the following would you do immediately following the initial assessment?

A. Obtain a thorough medical history.

B. Place the patient in the ambulance.

C. Ascertain the amount of time the patient has been gone.

D. Obtain a thorough set of vital signs.

20. Which of the following represent structures found in the upper airway?

A. nose, oropharynx, hypopharynx, vocal cords

B. nasopharynx, oropharynx, hypopharynx, larynx

C. nose, nasopharynx, oropharynx, hypopharynx

D. nasopharynx, hypopharynx, oropharynx, vocal cords

21. Your partner has intubated an unresponsive female with an endotracheal tube. After approximately 1 minute of positive pressure ventilation with a bag-valve-mask, she begins to groan loudly. What should your next action be?

A. Restrain the patient and continue positive pressure ventilation.

B. Assist the patient in her respiratory efforts.

C. Leave the endotracheal tube in place without positive pressure ventilation.

D. Check the tube placement.

22. Which of the following partially describes the mechanics of inhalation?

A. Contraction of the diaphragm decreases pressure in the lungs.

B. Relaxation of the diaphragm increases pressure in the lungs.

C. Contraction of the diaphragm increases pressure in the lungs.

D. Relaxation of the diaphragm decreases pressure in the lungs.

23. The structure that surrounds the external surface of the lung is the:

A. thoracic wall.

B. pleura.

C. diaphragm.

D. alveoli.

24. During normal respiration, which of the following best describes the physical principle responsible for the exchange of oxygen and carbon dioxide at the alveolar-capillary level?

A. difference in intrapulmonary pressure

B. changes in pulmonary volume

C. diffusion from a higher to a lower concentration

D. alveolar-capillary pressure differences

25. While assessing a combative 23-year-old male who has been stabbed in the right hemithorax you note he is dyspneic and cyanotic. Your immediate concern is:
    A. determining wound depth.
    B. assessing for a rib fracture.
    C. replacing lost fluid.
    D. managing the hypoxia.

26. What type of ventilation device provides the greatest tidal volume during positive pressure ventilation?
    A. mouth-to-pocket mask
    B. demand valve resuscitation
    C. bag-valve-mask
    D. nonrebreathing oxygen mask

27. You intubate an unresponsive 23-year-old male with a combitube airway. The patient has been shot in the back of the mouth and has profuse bleeding. After passing a combitube, you note equality in chest rise and fall and breath sounds. How would you continue airway management?
    A. Continue ventilating at a rate of 12–20 ventilations per minute.
    B. Extubate the patient and continue ventilating with a bag-valve-mask.
    C. Continue ventilations with a demand valve resuscitator.
    D. Extubate the patient and reattempt the intubation.

28. A patient has been struck by a car and continues to bleed from an open wound to the deformed right leg. Which of the following in addition to direct pressure, would control this hemorrhage best?
    A. splinting the right leg
    B. administering oxygen and elevating the extremity
    C. applying an ice pack to the bleeding area

D. placing the patient in a Trendelenburg position

29. An individual's mental status can be easily determined during the initial assessment by which of the following?
    A. directly observing whether or not the patient is talking
    B. a description as to whether the patient is semiconscious or coherent
    C. a mini-neurological exam using the AVPU method
    D. the level of consciousness is not ascertained during the initial assessment.

30. Which of the following best describes the Glasgow Coma Scale?
    A. a scale related to eye, verbal, and sensory function
    B. a quantification as to exact patient injury
    C. a numerical system to identify trends in the neurologic status of the patient
    D. a system that dictates what interventions the EMT-Intermediate must initiate

31. You are treating a patient whose chief complaint is lethargy and general malaise. At a minimum, what laboratory blood samples should be obtained prior to administering IV fluid?
    A. one red top and one green top blood tube
    B. one red top blood tube
    C. one green top and one gray top blood tube
    D. no samples are required

32. You are immobilizing a 32-year-old female onto a backboard. The patient has fallen down a flight of stairs and has suffered a large laceration to the frontal region of her head. The patient is on the backboard and manual spinal stabilization is being held.

What is the **best** order to apply the backboard straps?

A. legs, torso, head

B. torso, legs, head

C. head, torso, legs

D. torso, legs, no strap for the head because of the laceration

33. An elderly female who refused your treatment after falling and striking her head has died from a cerebral hemorrhage. Your best protection in this situation is:

A. the witness testimony of your partner.

B. the verbal report you gave your supervisor following the refusal.

C. a written narrative attached to a standard refusal form.

D. none—the standard refusal form is adequate.

34. You are called to a factory to treat three unconscious employees who were overcome by fumes. They are still in the building. How should you proceed at the scene?

A. Immediately enter the building and retrieve the patients.

B. Park the ambulance upwind from the factory and wait for the fire department.

C. Park the ambulance downwind from the factory and enter the building with oxygen on.

D. Prevent escape of additional fumes by closing all windows.

35. You are called to the scene of a shooting. The patient has been shot in the abdomen. You see the assailant as you approach the scene. You should:

A. immediately approach the injured person for treatment.

B. confront the person with the gun so you can begin treatment of the patient.

C. keep your ambulance at a safe distance and wait while your dispatcher calls for police assistance.

D. park the ambulance between the patient and the assailant and approach the patient.

36. You arrive on the scene of an unconscious multiple system trauma patient. You realize the need for paramedic backup. The best way to proceed would be to:

A. perform an initial assessment, extricate, and wait for paramedic backup.

B. perform an initial assessment, extricate, transport, start an IV, and meet paramedic backup en route.

C. perform an initial assessment, extricate, meet paramedic backup en route.

D. extricate, initial assessment, initiate an IV, disregard paramedic backup.

37. A patient has been struck in the anterior neck with a baseball. The patient is dyspneic and unable to speak. You would suspect an injury to what structure?

A. oropharynx

B. esophagus

C. larynx

D. the temporal lobe

38. Steam burns with secondary edema would be most concerning if it involved what structure?

A. hands

B. oropharynx

C. chest

D. arms

39. You are called to the scene of a car/pedestrian crash. The pedestrian was thrown to the side of the road. What airway maneuver would be most appropriate for this patient?
   A. endotracheal intubation
   B. head tilt-chin lift
   C. jaw thrust
   D. a manual airway maneuver is not needed

40. You are called to a restaurant for a man who is choking. When you arrive the patient is unconscious and lying on the floor. You establish unresponsiveness and open the airway. After an attempt to ventilate, the airway is still obstructed. What should be your next action?
   A. give five abdominal thrusts
   B. give five chest thrusts
   C. perform a finger sweep, then five abdominal thrusts
   D. reposition the head and attempt to ventilate

41. While ventilating a 73-year-old cardiac arrest patient, you are having difficulty maintaining the seal between the patient's face and the mask of the bag-valve-mask. You should:
   A. insert an oropharyngeal airway.
   B. remove the patient's dentures.
   C. change to a pocket mask.
   D. secure the mask to the face with tape.

42. As you are ventilating your patient with a bag-valve-mask, you note minimal bag resistance and rapid emptying. This would be associated with:
   A. an airway obstruction.
   B. normal ventilations.
   C. a mask leak.
   D. a hole in the bag.

43. You are ventilating an intubated patient with a bag-valve-mask, with supplemental oxygen connected to a reservoir. All of the following are signs of effective ventilation, **except**:
   A. equal chest rise and fall.
   B. bilateral breath sounds.
   C. abdominal distension.
   D. decrease in cyanosis.

44. You are treating a patient from a car crash. You suspect he is suffering from decreased perfusion. The patient's skin most likely will be:
   A. warm and dry.
   B. cool and pale.
   C. warm and pale.
   D. red and hot.

45. You are attending to an elderly male who lacerated his right forearm with an axe. He informs you that the accident occurred 2 hours ago and he immediately applied a tourniquet. The distal extremity is now deeply discolored and all bleeding has stopped. You would:
   A. remove the tourniquet to restore distal circulation.
   B. loosen the tourniquet slightly to restore distal circulation and replace after 5 minutes.
   C. gradually loosen the tourniquet so as to gradually restore distal circulation.
   D. leave the tourniquet in place and transport.

46. During the middle of winter you respond to a call where a 60-year-old female has been hit by a car. The patient is unresponsive. How should you proceed with your treatment?
   A. Perform the initial assessment, expose the patient, and do the rapid trauma assessment on scene.

B. Establish responsiveness, perform the initial assessment, expose the patient, and continue with the rapid trauma assessment on scene.

C. Perform the initial assessment and immobilization on scene. Expose the patient and continue the rapid trauma assessment in the ambulance.

D. Perform the initial assessment and rapid trauma assessment. Exposing the patient is not necessary.

47. You are transporting a 65-year-old female who has fractured her right hip in a fall. During your reassessment of the patient, what information would be most important?

A. allergies the patient may have

B. complaint of nausea

C. the severity of the pain

D. presence or absence of a distal pulse

48. You are treating an elderly male patient who fell and has a possible hip fracture. The patient tells you he was dizzy before he fell. How should you prepare this patient for transport?

A. Packaging includes immobilization only.

B. Packaging is complete once you finish the initial assessment.

C. Packaging should include fracture stabilization and transport.

D. Packaging should include complete spinal immobilization and fracture stabilization.

49. Which statement is most accurate about securing a patient to the cot?

A. The patient only needs to be secured to the cot when the ambulance is moving.

B. There should be a minimum of four straps holding the patient to the cot.

C. If the patient is secured to the backboard, it is not necessary to secure the patient to the cot.

D. The patient should be secured to the cot before transfer to the ambulance.

50. You are treating a 60-year-old male complaining of chest discomfort. The family wants the patient transported to a hospital in the next town which is 12 miles away. While en route, the patient's condition starts to deteriorate and his mental status decreases. What should be your next decision?

A. Continue transport to the facility of family choice.

B. Call the family for permission to take the patient to a closer hospital.

C. Transport the patient to the closest hospital for stabilization.

D. Speed up your transportation to the facility in the next town.

51. The primary purpose of performing an initial assessment is:

A. to determine if rapid transport is necessary.

B. to determine if a BLS unit can transport this patient without tying up an Intermediate Life Support unit.

C. to manage life threats and establish priorities of care.

D. to determine vital signs.

52. Which of the following hazards are you most likely to encounter at a medical emergency?

A. broken glass

B. infectious pathogens

C. risk of fire

D. confined spaces

53. You are dispatched to a motor vehicle crash that requires using extrication tools to free the patient. In addition to ensuring your safety, you should:
    A. park your vehicle downwind to avoid any hazardous materials.
    B. provide protection for your patient with a blanket or similar device.
    C. ask the tool operator to stay away from the patient's side of the vehicle.
    D. notify medical control that there may be additional injuries from the extrication.

54. All of the following are elements of the initial assessment, **except**:
    A. checking carotid and radial pulses.
    B. assessing the skin color, temperature, and condition.
    C. assessing the volume of inspired breaths.
    D. checking the patient's vital signs.

55. Identify the order of anatomical structures which serves as the route air takes when traveling from the mouth to the trachea.
    1. vocal cords
    2. cricoid cartilage
    3. oropharynx
    4. epiglottis
    5. glottic opening

    A. 3, 4, 5, 1, 2
    B. 3, 5, 4, 2, 1
    C. 4, 3, 5, 2, 1
    D. 4, 3, 2, 5, 1

56. The nasal cavity performs all the following functions, **except**:
    A. warming air that enters to body temperature.
    B. excreting mucus to prevent excess dehumidification.
    C. filtering air that enters by turbulent precipitation.

D. humidifying 100 percent of air that enters.

57. Which of the following would be most likely to cause an airway obstruction?
    A. pulmonary edema
    B. epiglotittis
    C. laryngitis
    D. acute bronchitis

58. The diffusion of oxygen into the capillary and carbon dioxide out of the capillary occurs at the:
    A. alveolar-capillary membrane.
    B. visceral-pleural membrane.
    C. alveolar-tissue membrane.
    D. tissue-capillary membrane.

59. Hypoxia, caused by something other than a direct ventilation disturbance, occurs in which of the following?
    A. epiglotittis
    B. pneumonia
    C. pneumothorax
    D. pulmonary embolism

60. Which of the following is the preferred method of ventilating a non-breathing patient?
    A. one-person bag-valve-mask
    B. two-person bag-valve-mask
    C. mouth-to-mask
    D. flow-restricted, oxygen powered ventilation device

61. Which of the following is a sign of inadequate ventilation?
    A. The heart rate begins to decrease.
    B. Gastric distention develops.
    C. The SpO_2 reading increases.
    D. The skin color becomes less cyanotic.

62. Which of the following would be appropriate when suctioning?
    A. Use only a rigid tonsil-tip catheter to suction.
    B. Apply suction while slowly removing the catheter.
    C. Set the suction at no more than -60 mmHg.
    D. Apply suction while slowly inserting the catheter for 15 seconds.

63. A mini-neurological exam can be conducted using the following mnemonic:
    A. SAMPLE
    B. PQRST-A
    C. AVPU
    D. APGAR

64. You have been dispatched to the home of a 17-year-old female who was injured while playing soccer. She is complaining of leg pain. Her father states that sometime during the game he saw her get hit in the shin by another player's foot. Which of the following would **not** be part of the initial assessment?
    A. asking her name and how old she is
    B. checking her radial pulses
    C. evaluating her skin condition, color and temperature
    D. exposing and palpating the lower extremity

65. All of the following are benefits of drawing a blood sample for the hospital prior to initiating an IV line, **except**:
    A. obtaining blood glucose levels.
    B. typing and cross-matching.
    C. determining baseline chemistries.
    D. determining the proteinuria levels.

66. You are called to the scene of a motor vehicle crash. Upon arrival, you find a 30-year-old male who was the unrestrained driver. Your initial assessment reveals that he is unresponsive; radial pulse is absent, carotid pulse is rapid and weak, respirations are about 42/minute and shallow. You note a contusion on the chest that approximates the steering wheel. Your priorities for managing this patient include:
    A. take in-line spinal stabilization, insert an oropharyngeal airway, and begin positive pressure ventilation.
    B. take in-line spinal stabilization, apply a nonrebreather mask at 15 lpm.
    C. insert an oropharyngeal airway, begin bag-valve-mask ventilation, and apply the PASG.
    D. take in-line spinal stabilization, begin bag-valve-mask ventilation, and start two large-bore IVs of normal saline.

67. You have responded to the scene of a motorcycle versus car crash. Your patient was the motorcycle rider, who was thrown 30 feet from the bike. His injuries include an open skull fracture with brain matter exposed, oral trauma with blood and broken teeth in the mouth, chest trauma resulting in a left thoracic flail segment, and bilateral femur fractures. His vitals are BP 92/60, HR 128, RR 40 and shallow. After taking in-line spinal stabilization, your next treatment priority is to:
    A. perform a head tilt-chin lift and begin bag-valve-mask ventilation.
    B. suction the mouth and begin positive pressure ventilation with O_2.
    C. suction the oropharynx and apply a nonrebreather mask at 15 lpm.
    D. stabilize the flail segment.

68. Of the following assessments or interventions, which one would be performed last during the rapid trauma assessment of an unresponsive patient with severe head, face, and neck trauma?

    A. auscultation of breath sounds

    B. palpation of the head

    C. palpation of the thorax

    D. application of the cervical spinal immobilization collar

69. You arrive on the scene of a tractor-trailer rollover which has pinned the male driver under the rig. As you approach the driver, you notice a placard on the trailer denoting its contents as flammable. You should immediately:

    A. continue to the patient's side and begin your assessment.

    B. quickly scan the trailer for leaks, if none noted, proceed.

    C. stop and call for the fire department.

    D. retreat and leave the scene.

70. During extrication of a patient trapped in an automobile, the fire department prepares to cut off the roof. Which of the following will provide the best protection to the patient during the procedure?

    A. stay outside the auto and instruct the patient to lie still

    B. stay inside the auto and place a thick blanket over both of you

    C. stay outside the auto and place a flame-retardant blanket over the patient

    D. stay inside the auto and place protective eyewear on the patient

71. In an unresponsive patient, the tongue may fall posteriorly and occlude the airway at what anatomic site?

    A. oropharynx

    B. carina

    C. nasopharynx

    D. laryngopharynx

72. Which of the following is **not** a physiological function of the mucous membranes covering the nasal conchae?

    A. warm the air

    B. entrap foreign material in air

    C. humidify the inspired air

    D. perceive the sense of smell

73. You have just placed an oropharyngeal airway in an unresponsive patient. In order to ensure a patient airway, you must also:

    A. perform the head tilt-chin lift maneuver.

    B. insert a gastric levine tube to decompress the stomach.

    C. use the two-hand BVM technique.

    D. apply oxygen tubing to the pocket mask.

74. What is the major pathophysiologic change that occurs with a simple pneumothorax?

    A. loss of perfusion around the alveoli

    B. loss of negative pressure in the pleural space

    C. loss of diaphragmatic function

    D. loss of phrenic nerve innervation

75. Which of the following properly describes how to secure a pocket mask to the face when performing mouth-to-mask ventilations?

    A. Place one hand around the top portion of the mask and apply pressure downward to ensure an adequate seal.

    B. Encircle both hands around the top portion of the mask and apply pressure downward to ensure an adequate seal.

    C. Place your thumbs along each side of the mask using your palms to push downward while lifting the mandible with your fingers to help ensure a good seal.

D. Place your thumbs under the mandible and lift while holding the mask in place with your fingers and use your palms to ensure a good seal.

76. Which of the following would indicate the need for immediate positive pressure ventilation?
A. a pulse oximeter (SpO_2) reading of 89 percent
B. a respiratory rate of 30 with adequate chest rise and fall
C. peripheral cyanosis
D. a respiratory rate of 24 with shallow depth

77. The heart contains a group of specialized cells which can initiate an impulse. These cells are known to have the property of:
A. automaticity.
B. conductivity.
C. contractility.
D. excitability.

78. You are treating a patient with an open upper right leg fracture with spurting blood. Which anatomic structure is probably responsible for the bleeding?
A. femoral artery
B. tibial artery
C. iliac artery
D. femoral vein

79. Of the following, which would be found through the process of inspection during the assessment?
A. crepitus to the left hemithorax
B. bilateral wheezing
C. hyperresonance to right hemithorax
D. paradoxical movement to right thorax

80. You are treating a patient who fell 30 feet off a scaffold. The patient is responsive but is complaining of severe pain to his back and neck. The patient also has a puncture wound to the abdomen. His arms are cool and moist while his legs are warm and dry, capillary refill is delayed, pupils are reactive to light, abdomen is soft to palpation. His vitals are BP 86/50, HR is 60, RR is 18. The patient is most likely suffering from:
A. vasogenic shock.
B. ruptured aortic artery.
C. myocardial contusion.
D. hypovolemic shock.

81. Of the following interventions, which should be delayed until you are en route to the hospital when treating a trauma victim?
A. applying a non-rebreather at 15 lpm
B. dressing and bandaging all wounds.
C. applying a cervical spinal immobilization collar
D. applying a traction splint

82. Which of the following is performed last when immobilizing a patient to a backboard?
A. assess pulse, motor, and sensory function
B. apply cervical spinal immobilization collar
C. secure the legs to the board
D. apply a head immobilization device

83. You are reassessing a patient while en route to the hospital. During this phase of patient assessment, which one of the following injuries should already have been managed?
A. puncture wound to the left thigh
B. foreign body in the eye
C. right humerus protruding through skin
D. open wound to the posterior thorax

84. List the following in order according to priority care performed on the patient.
    1. control bleeding from a small laceration
    2. initiate bag-valve-mechanical ventilation
    3. assess the carotid pulse
    4. perform a jaw thrust

    A. 1, 2, 3, 4
    B. 4, 2, 1, 3
    C. 4, 2, 3, 1
    D. 2, 4, 3, 1

85. Which of the following hazards would you be least concerned with during the scene size-up?
    A. blood spurting from an open soft tissue injury
    B. an extremely cold home in the winter
    C. a hostile crowd at an accident scene
    D. extremely hot pavement

86. Which of the following would be **incorrect** regarding scene size-up?
    A. Consider all power lines to be energized at a crash scene.
    B. Delay entry to a hostile scene until arrival of an additional EMS unit.
    C. Do not enter water to perform a rescue unless specially trained to do so.
    D. Assume confined spaces contain toxic substances or are low oxygen areas.

87. Which technique listed below is most effective in controlling the crowd at the scene of an emergency?
    A. Assign two EMT-Intermediates to provide crowd control.
    B. Have the patient's family members stand around the patient.

C. Contact the police to control the scene.
D. Involve crowd members for crowd control.

88. Additional resources that are commonly required to assess emergency scenes include all of the following, **except**:
    A. law enforcement.
    B. fire/rescuer resources.
    C. electric utility.
    D. coroner's investigation.

89. The following list pairs common classifications of emergencies with a description. Which items are **incorrectly** paired?
    A. medical—illness
    B. behavioral—abnormal behavior
    C. gynecology—childbirth
    D. trauma—injury

90. The first step in the initial assessment is to assess the
    A. breathing rate and depth.
    B. airway patency.
    C. presence of a pulse.
    D. general impression.

91. Which statement most correctly describes the purpose of performing the initial assessment?
    A. identify all injuries and treat them as found.
    B. identify all potential threats to life first, then manage them according to priority.
    C. evaluate clinical findings and vital signs
    D. identify immediate life threats and manage them as they are found.

92. Which of the following structures is superior to the pharynx?
    A. angle of Louis

B. nasopharynx

C. carina

D. laryngopharynx

93. Which airway management method is **incorrectly** paired with description?

A. head tilt-chin lift—displaces the jaw forward and extends the head

B. chin lift—pulls the chin forward displacing the tongue.

C. jaw thrust—extends the head and moves the mandible forward.

D. airway adjunct—displaces the tongue away from the posterior oropharynx

94. You are dispatched to a local restaurant. You arrive on scene and observe a 40-year-old patient clutching his throat and coughing forcefully. You should immediately:

A. deliver repeated abdominal thrusts until the obstruction is removed.

B. encourage the patient to continue to cough.

C. insert a laryngoscope and remove the object with Magill forceps.

D. perform a tongue-jaw lift and attempt to ventilate.

95. The preferred method to maintain an airway in the suspected spine injured patient is the:

A. head tilt-chin lift.

B. chin lift.

C. jaw thrust.

D. nasopharyngeal airway.

96. The level at which the trachea divides into the right and left mainstream bronchus is the:

A. terminal alveoli.

B. alveolar duct.

C. carina.

D. cricoid.

97. Which of the following best describes the layers of thorax from the outermost to the innermost?

A. thoracic wall, parietal pleura, pleural space, visceral pleura

B. thoracic wall, pleural space, parietal pleura, visceral pleura

C. thoracic wall, visceral pleura, parietal pleura, pleural space

D. thoracic wall, visceral pleura, pleural space, parietal pleura

98. Which statement best describes the mechanical process of inhalation?

A. diaphragm relaxes, intrathoracic pressure is lower than atmospheric air pressure

B. diaphragm contracts, intercostal muscles contract, intrathoracic pressure is greater than atmospheric air pressure

C. diaphragm does not move, intercostal muscles relax, intrathoracic pressure is lower than atmospheric air pressure

D. diaphragm contracts, intercostal muscles contract, intrathoracic pressure is lower than atmospheric air pressure

99. Which statement best describes the mechanical process of exhalation?

A. diaphragm moves up, intercostal muscles contract, intrathoracic pressure is lower than atmospheric air pressure

B. diaphragm moves up, intercostal muscles relax, intrathoracic pressure is greater than atmospheric air pressure

C. diaphragm does not move, intrathoracic pressure is lower than atmospheric air pressure

D. diaphragm moves down, intercostal muscles relax, intrathoracic pressure is lower than atmospheric air pressure

100. Which statement best describes the process of gas exchange across a capillary membrane?
    A. gases move from an area of higher concentration to an area of lower concentration
    B. gases move from an area of lower concentration to an area of high concentration
    C. gases do not move across the alveolar-capillary membrane
    D. gases move from areas of equal concentrations

101. Which cardiovascular structure is **incorrectly** paired with its description?
    A. epicardium—the innermost layer of the heart
    B. pericardium—sac that surrounds the heart
    C. apex—the lower border of the heart
    D. mitral valve—valve between the left atrium and left ventricle

102. What is typically the **earliest** detectable clinical sign of decreased blood volume?
    A. increased heart rate
    B. increased cardiac stroke volume
    C. peripheral vasoconstriction
    D. diaphoresis

103. If the radial pulse is absent because of poor perfusion, which of the following other pulses would you suspect would also be absent?
    A. carotid pulse
    B. femoral pulse
    C. apical pulse
    D. dorsalis pedis pulse

104. To ensure adequate ventilation with an esophageal obturator airway (EOA), you must:
    A. frequently check the status of the inflation balloon on the distal end of the esophageal obturator airway.
    B. maintain the head and neck in a neutral position.
    C. inflate the distal balloon with 10 ccs of air.
    D. maintain an airtight seal between the patient's face and the esophageal obturator airway mask.

105. After intubating the patient with an endotracheal tube, to check for proper placement you must:
    A. ventilate the patient for one minute before auscultating breath sounds.
    B. attach the pulse oximeter and check the reading.
    C. ventilate the patient and auscultate over the epigastrium then each hemithorax.
    D. check for condensation in the ET tube with each ventilation.

106. Which of the following is true regarding endotracheal suctioning?
    A. To determine the catheter length, measure from the lips to the ear lobe.
    B. Insert the catheter down the endotracheal tube with suction applied.
    C. Advance the catheter to the level of the carina.
    D. Apply suction for at least 20 seconds.

107. Hypoperfusion or shock is described as inadequate:
    A. fraction of inspired oxygen.
    B. removal of carbon dioxide from the alveolar tissue.

C. levels of hemoglobin that prevent the movement of oxygen from the blood plasma.

D. delivery of oxygen and elimination of carbon dioxide from cells.

108. Physiologically unstable patients should be reassessed every:

A. 5 minutes.

B. 10 minutes.

C. 15 minutes.

D. 20 minutes.

109. You are dispatched to a patient who has been stabbed in the neck. You observe a responsive patient in obvious respiratory distress. His neck appears to be swollen, and you feel crepitation upon palpatation. This finding is described as:

A. pericardial tamponade.

B. subcutaneous emphysema.

C. tension pneumothorax.

D. hematoma.

110. The parameters evaluated in the revised trauma score are:

A. respiratory effort, diastolic blood pressure, and Glasgow Coma Score.

B. respiratory rate, diastolic blood pressure, and Glasgow Coma Score.

C. respiratory effort, systolic blood pressure, and Glasgow Coma Score.

D. respiratory rate, systolic blood pressure, and Glasgow Coma Score.

111. Which of the following is least important when initially taking a patient history?

A. the patient's last oral intake

B. the patient's allergies

C. the patient's father's medical history

D. radiation of pain to another body region

112. Which of the following is **not** a laboratory test routinely performed by the hospital on prehospital blood samples?

A. human immunodeficiency virus

B. blood glucose

C. complete blood count

D. type and cross-match

113. Which of the following is true regarding reassessment of the patient?

A. It is performed to detect changes in the patient's condition, assess other complaints, and to guide continued care.

B. It is a complete head-to-toe physical exam repeated every 5 or 15 minutes.

C. Reassessment of patients during transport should be conducted only if time or the patient's condition permits it.

D. It is an assessment of the airway, breathing, and circulation that is performed every 30 minutes.

114. The most important factor to consider when determining the appropriate medical facility to transport the patient to is based on the:

A. patient's choice.

B. closest in distance.

C. patient's condition.

D. patient's physician.

115. Which statement best describes the potential results from using lights and siren while transporting a patient?

A. Patient care is improved dramatically by the use of lights and siren.

B. Patient care is distracted by the use of lights and siren.

C. Patients typically request lights and sirens and are calmed by their use.

D. Accidents occur less frequently when using lights and siren.

116. An order you receive from medical direction appears to be improper. Select the statement that best describes the action to be taken.
    A. Follow the order without question.
    B. Follow the order and then document it carefully.
    C. Repeat the orders, as given, back to medical control.
    D. Follow the order and consult with medical direction once at the hospital.

117. The ongoing assessment should always include reassessment of which of the following items?
    A. initial assessment
    B. focused physical exam
    C. detailed history
    D. detailed physical exam

118. Scene safety begins:
    A. with the call received from the dispatch center.
    B. once you approach the scene at that location.
    C. after exiting the vehicle.
    D. while visualizing the scene by walking the perimeter.

119. Your unit is the first on scene of a serious vehicle crash. You notice that wires are lying across the roof of the vehicle. You should:
    A. stage outside the scene and call for specially trained personnel.
    B. carefully approach the vehicle by shuffling your feet and quickly gain entry through a window.
    C. cut the wire closest to the pole.
    D. cautiously remove the wires by using a wooden or fiberglass pole.

120. You are at the scene of a fight when a group of bystanders suddenly become hostile and threatening. You should:
    A. try to reason with the group so that you can continue to provide treatment.
    B. quietly call for police, continue care, and protect the patient.
    C. immediately leave the scene until it is secured.
    D. clear the crowd by using necessary force.

121. While approaching a vehicle crash site, you are unsure what level of body substance isolation (BSI) precautions you will need. You should at least:
    A. apply gloves, protective eyewear, and a HEPA mask.
    B. assess the scene further, and then decide what is needed.
    C. use gloves and return to your vehicle if other BSI is necessary.
    D. use gloves and eye protection.

122. You are treating a patient in a busy department store. Which of the following is the best way to protect the patient from the gaze of the public?
    A. Ask the bystanders to leave the scene or you will be forced to have then removed.
    B. Have your partner hold a blanket up with outstretched arms to block their view.
    C. Have the bystanders turn their backs to the patient while holding an unfolded sheet.
    D. Shield the patient from the curious bystanders by placing the stretcher between them.

123. You arrive on a scene of a multiple vehicle crash and find eight critically injured patients. Only three ambulances are immediately available. Your next immediate action should be to:

A. divide the critically injured patients and transport immediately.

B. initiate the multiple casualty incident plan.

C. quickly treat all immediate life threats first, then move to other injuries.

D. immediately transport the most critical patient.

124. You find your patient standing on the roof of a vehicle that is partially submerged in fast-moving water. You should immediately:

A. call for personnel who are specially trained in water rescue.

B. form a human chain with bystanders and assist the patient to shore.

C. throw the patient a rope and ask him or her to hold on, then pull the patient to safety.

D. tie a rescue rope to yourself and make an attempt to reach the patient.

125. You are dispatched to a female patient complaining of respiratory difficulty. The scene size-up does not reveal any unusual situations or hazards. A bystander states that the patient has had this problem before. From this information, you would initially categorize the patient's problem as:

A. trauma.

B. behavioral.

C. medical.

D. obstetric.

126. Which of the following upper-airway structures warms and filters inspired air?

A. mucous membrane

B. inferior turbinate

C. superior conchae

D. external nares

127. Stridor is caused by:

A. presence of fluids in the upper airway.

B. constriction of the bronchioles.

C. tracheal obstruction.

D. laryngeal edema.

128. The Magill forceps may be used in conjunction with _____ to remove an airway obstruction.

A. four back blows

B. direct laryngoscopy

C. index finger sweeps

D. oropharyngeal airway

129. After you have inserted an oropharyngeal airway, the patient begins to gag. You should:

A. turn the patient on his or her side.

B. prepare to suction the airway.

C. quickly remove the airway.

D. immediately coach the patient to relax.

130. You are preparing to insert a nasopharyngeal airway. You should:

A. lubricate it with a water soluble lubricant and insert it at a 45-degree lateral angle to the septum.

B. lubricate it with a petroleum jelly and insert the airway into the more patent nostril.

C. lubricate it with a water soluble lubricant and insert it with the bevel towards the septum.

D. lubricate it with a petroleum lubricant and insert it in the right nostril only.

131. You are treating an unresponsive adult patient involved in a vehicle crash. As you perform the initial assessment you hear sonorous sounds. You should immediately:

A. do a head tilt-chin lift and hold in-line stabilization.

B. suction and continue with the assessment.

C. apply Sellick's maneuver and begin bag-valve-mask ventilation.

D. do a jaw thrust and insert an oropharyngeal airway.

132. Which of the following is **not** an initial sign of suspected spine injury?
    A. pale, cool, clammy skin below the site of injury
    B. diaphragmatic breathing
    C. priaprism
    D. loss of sensation in lower extremities

133. Oxygen (O_2) and carbon dioxide (CO_2) gas exchange occurs in the:
    A. alveolar ducts.
    B. pleura.
    C. terminal bronchioles.
    D. alveoli.

134. All of the statements regarding the bag-valve-mask are true, **except**:
    A. tidal volumes delivered by bag-valve-mask are less than those delivered by pocket mask.
    B. two rescuers are recommended when using the bag-valve-mask.
    C. the bag-valve-mask is the recommended device to use when only one person is available to ventilate.
    D. nearly 100 percent oxygen concentration can be delivered by bag-valve-mask when using a reservoir.

135. Which of the following may indicate inadequate ventilation?
    A. Heart rate decreases from 124 to 100 per minute.
    B. Chest rises with each ventilation.
    C. Patient's skin is warm, dry, and pink.
    D. Pop-off valve releases air with each ventilation.

136. All of the following may result from decreased perfusion, **except**:
    A. cells will begin to move from aerobic to anaerobic metabolism.
    B. glucose metabolism will produce lactic acid.
    C. cell death may result from the accumulation of acids.
    D. pyruvic acid breaks down into carbon dioxide and water.

137. Which of the following is the leading cause of cardiac arrest and sudden death?
    A. coronary artery disease
    B. acid-base imbalance
    C. cerebrovascular accident
    D. pulmonary embolism

138. Which of the following is the most reliable indicator of poor perfusion in the adult patient?
    A. pale, cool, clammy skin
    B. capillary refill that is less than 2 seconds
    C. skin that is cool to the touch
    D. constricted pupils that are brisk to respond to light.

139. You arrive on the scene and find a 23-year-old male patient who was stabbed in the chest. Upon your assessment you find blood in the mouth, and a respiratory rate of 42 and shallow. You should immediately:
    A. assess the radial and carotid pulse.
    B. obtain a set of baseline vital signs.
    C. administer oxygen by non-rebreather at 15 lpm.
    D. suction the mouth and begin bag-valve-mask ventilation.

140. You have responded to the scene of a serious motor vehicle crash. While performing the rapid trauma assessment, you should:
    A. remove all jewelry.
    B. manage non-life-threatening bleeding.
    C. dress all wounds.
    D. expose the patient.

141. In which circumstance should you **not** expose the patient to perform an assessment?

   A. in an environment that may lead to hypothermia

   B. a motor vehicle crash in which the patient was ejected

   C. if a crowd has gathered at the scene

   D. if your partner is treating another patient

142. The most reliable component of the ongoing assessment to reassess in the head-injured patient to identify deterioration or improvement in the patient's condition is:

   A. the blood pressure.

   B. pupil reactivity to light.

   C. the skin.

   D. the mental status.

143. Which assessment or management technique is **not** a part of the detailed physical exam?

   A. application of a cervical spinal immobilization collar

   B. palpating for abdominal masses and rigidity

   C. inspecting the sclera for icterus

   D. auscultation of breath sounds

144. Your patient has fallen approximately 20 feet onto a concrete floor. While palpating the chest you feel a crackling sensation at the upper chest and base of the neck. You can best describe this as:

   A. a flail segment.

   B. subcutaneous emphysema.

   C. paradoxical motion.

   D. suprasternal notch reaction.

145. The GCS evaluates all of the following parameters **except**:

   A. eye opening.

   B. respiratory rate/minute.

   C. best verbal response.

   D. best motor response.

146. Which is **incorrect** regarding the use and securing of the portable cot?

   A. When using the pole cot, it is preferable to use four rescuers.

   B. Canvas cots alone should not be used to support a spinal injury.

   C. Portable cots should be loaded prior to the wheeled cot.

   D. These are not recommended for patients weighing more than 250 pounds.

147. In which of the following would emergency care be conducted after the removal of the patient from a vehicle?

   A. The patient is not oriented and not cooperating.

   B. There will be a delay in extrication.

   C. The vehicle is on its side and unstable.

   D. The patient complains of cervical pain.

148. During transport the patient begins to complain of abdominal pain. You should:

   A. increase the oxygen flow.

   B. perform a complete detailed physical exam.

   C. administer nitro to the patient.

   D. perform a focused assessment of the area of the complaint.

149. Which physical findings would cause you to categorize the patient as a priority?

   A. BP 100/60, pulse 82, R13 and normal

   B. side impact in a motor vehicle collision

   C. Glasgow Coma Score less than 9

   D. open humerus fracture

150. The purpose of providing a brief, concise, relevant oral report to the hospital staff when transferring care is:
    A. that it is a requirement of the hospital staff to receive a report from EMS.
    B. to provide the hospital staff the legal right to treat the patient.
    C. to ensure a continuation of care.
    D. to avoid being charged with negligence.

151. Which statement regarding the prehospital care report is **not** true?
    A. The report will prevent you from being sued.
    B. You should use a standardized format.
    C. Reports become a permanent part of the patient's medical records.
    D. Your report becomes your best legal defense in a court of law.

152. You arrive on the scene and find a 23-year-old male patient who was involved in a fight. Upon your initial assessment you find blood in the mouth and tachypnea that is shallow and labored. The skin is extremely pale, cyanotic, and diaphoretic. Your next immediate action is to:
    A. suction the mouth and apply a non-rebreather at 15 lpm.
    B. take in-line immobilization, suction, and begin positive pressure ventilation.
    C. expose the patient to inspect for open wounds to the thorax.
    D. check the radial pulse and capillary refill, then apply a nonrebreather mask at 15 lpm.

153. You arrive on the scene of a patient complaining of severe crushing substernal chest pain. As you approach the patient, he states "I am having a difficult time breathing." Your next immediate action is to:

    A. perform a head tilt-chin lift and assess the tidal volume.
    B. assess breath sound and begin bag-valve-mask ventilation.
    C. assess the radial pulse and apply a non-rebreather mask.
    D. take a set of vitals and gather a SAMPLE history.

154. You open the airway of an unresponsive medical patient using a jaw thrust. The patient continues to produce sonorous sounds. You should immediately:
    A. begin bag-valve-mask ventilation.
    B. reposition the mandible using the jaw thrust.
    C. insert an endotracheal tube.
    D. assess the respiratory status.

155. Which of the following has been demonstrated to provide the greatest tidal volume during ventilation?
    A. combitube and bag-valve-mask
    B. mouth-to-mask ventilation
    C. one-person bag-valve-mask
    D. two-person bag-valve-mask

156. You arrive on the scene and find a male patient in his 30s lying supine on the street. There are no bystanders at the scene. He is not alert and appears grossly cyanotic. Your first immediate action is to:
    A. open the airway and begin bag-valve-mask ventilation.
    B. call for additional resources.
    C. take in-line immobilization and perform a jaw thrust.
    D. quickly scan the scene for any hazards.

157. Which of the following would not be discovered during the initial assessment of the patient?
    A. decreased minute ventilation

B. tachycardia

C. poor skin turgor

D. hypotension

158. During the spinal immobilzation process, you should ensure that:

A. the feet are strapped to the board.

B. a cervical collar is applied after the log-roll.

C. the head is secured after strapping the torso.

D. backboard straps are applied to the abdomen, and across the lower legs.

159. You arrive on the scene to find an alert 46-year-old female patient complaining of severe abdominal pain. You place the patient on a nonrebreather mask and assess the radial pulse and skin color, temperature, and condition. Your next immediate action is:

A. obtain a SAMPLE history, conduct a focused physical exam, and get a set of baseline vital signs.

B. start an IV of normal saline and obtain a set of vital signs.

C. perform a detailed physical exam and obtain a SAMPLE history.

D. prepare the patient for transport and conduct an initial assessment en route to the medical facility.

160. You are at the residence of a patient who is complaining of abdominal pain. The patient is stable at this time. Which of the following would guide your continued care?

A. orders from the patient's son who is a physician

B. your local protocol

C. orders from the family physician

D. the advice from your partner

161. You arrive on the scene and find an unresponsive elderly male patient in his bed. As you approach the patient you note snoring-type respirations. You should immediately:

A. insert an oropharyngeal airway.

B. insert a nasopharyngeal airway.

C. perform a head tilt-chin lift.

D. begin bag-valve-mask ventilation.

162. Adequate ventilation, when using an endotracheal tube, is best confirmed by:

A. an absence of gastric insufflation.

B. absence of cyanosis.

C. equal bilateral breath sounds in all lung fields.

D. absence of end tidal CO_2 production.

163. Which of the following best describes the exchange of gasses in the alveoli?

A. oxygen leaves the capillary and enters the alveoli.

B. carbon dioxide diffuses out of the alveoli and into the capillary.

C. carbon dioxide enters the capillary bed and attaches to hemoglobin.

D. oxygen diffuses out of the alveoli and enters the capillary.

164. Which of the following conditions would cause an obstructive type of shock?

A. congestive heart failure.

B. hemorrhage.

C. allergic reaction.

D. pericardial tamponade.

165. The following are true regarding the prehospital care report **except**:

A. it can be admissible as evidence in a court of law.

B. it may be used for quality assurance monitoring.

C. it is used by some EMS systems for billing purposes.

D. it does not become a part of the permanent patient record.

166. In which of the following patient presentations would obtaining a venous blood sample be most important?
    A. altered mental status with bizarre behavior
    B. acute onset of respiratory distress
    C. abdominal pain with specks of blood in the vomitus
    D. severe headache that is chronic in nature

167. You have a patient who is entrapped in a car whose fuel tank has ruptured and is burning. As efforts are expended to free the victim, what would best protect the patient from being harmed by the heat and flames?
    A. Place the patient in firefighter's turnout gear.
    B. Shield the patient with a short spine board.
    C. Cover the patient with a flame retardant blanket.
    D. Nothing can be done at this point for the patient.

168. A flail segment impairs adequate ventilation by:
    A. decreasing the effectiveness of thoracic movement.
    B. causing an upper airway obstruction.
    C. paralyzing the diaphragm.
    D. allowing air to collect in the pleural space.

169. Normal speech is produced when:
    A. air entering the lungs causes the vocal cords to vibrate.
    B. the pharynx changes its size due to muscular contractions.
    C. air exiting the lungs causing the vocal cords to vibrate.
    D. changes is tracheal diameter.

170. During the management of a patient in cardiac arrest, the major purpose for providing CPR is to:
    A. treat the underlying cause of cardiac arrest.
    B. provide artificial ventilation and circulation so that defibrillation and drug therapy can be provided.
    C. give the family hope all that can be done is being done.
    D. restore normal cardiac activity.

171. A 17-year-old vehicle crash victim sustained the following injuries. Which one of these would be treated during the detailed physical exam?
    A. an abdominal evisceration
    B. lacerations to the dorsum of the hand
    C. an open femur fracture
    D. knife wound to the posterior thorax

172. A patient cut her hand while peeling an apple with a paring knife. Which of the following would be most appropriate to control the bleeding?
    A. tourniquet applied to the forearm
    B. digital pressure on the radial artery
    C. digital pressure on the ulnar artery
    D. direct pressure to the site of injury

173. Two EMS units responding to the same call using lights and siren, traveling closely one behind the other is potentially dangerous because:
    A. there is a greater likelihood for motorists to panic and wreck.
    B. both sirens operating simultaneously may actually diminish the ability for other motorists to hear the approaching sirens.

C. a car may pull into traffic after the first unit passes assuming that the road is now safe to travel.

D. there is a greater risk for both units to get lost driving to the address since one usually follows the other.

174. You are summoned to a fast-food restaurant where someone is reportedly choking on chicken nuggets. Initial attempts to clear the airway by providing subdiaphgramatic thrusts have failed. As an EMT-I, you should now:

A. initiate transport to the hospital.

B. wait for the patient to go into cardiac arrest and then treat the patient as a cardiac arrest victim.

C. perform a visual laryngoscopy and retrieve the foreign object.

D. lay the patient on the ground and deliver sharp back blows.

175. What would be considered as appropriate body substance isolation when preparing to intubate?

A. gown, gloves

B. mask, gloves, eye protection

C. gloves only

D. gown, gloves, eye protection, mask

176. Disentangling a person from a car, or removing them from an awkward location in a home is generally known as patient _____.

A. extraction

B. extrication

C. removal

D. interaction

177. A person who is successfully intubated with an endotracheal tube cannot speak because:

A. the vocal cords cannot vibrate.

B. the BVM mask covers the face.

C. the delivery of PPV precludes the contraction of vocal cord muscles.

D. air is not passing over the cords during inspiration.

178. You are called for a patient who is complaining of chest pain and severe shortness of breath. Your first action upon arrival at the scene is to:

A. open the airway and assess the breathing status.

B. apply a nonrebreather at 15 lpm.

C. begin bag-valve-mask ventilation and check for a pulse.

D. assess the scene for safety hazards.

179. You are called to the scene of a possible shooting. When you arrive, the wife of the patient meets you at the curb and states the patient is bleeding profusely from a wound to the chest. You should immediately:

A. determine if the perpetrator is still on the scene.

B. stop the bleeding with direct pressure.

C. apply your gloved hand over the wound.

D. begin bag-valve-mask ventilation with supplemental oxygen.

180. You are called to the scene for a patient who is complaining of feeling ill for the last week. He has a fever, a cough with blood-tinged sputum, and shortness of breath. Before entering the scene, you should:

A. call for a backup in case it is a cardiac arrest.

B. put on gloves, eye protection, and a HEPA respirator.

C. contact medical direction for orders to treat the patient.

D. put on gloves and eye protection.

181. You are treating a patient at the scene of an auto crash at a busy intersection. A crowd gathers to see what is going on. As you conduct your physical assessment of the patient, it is necessary to:

A. disperse the crowd immediately.

B. move the ambulance between the crowd and the patient.

C. cover the patient with a sheet as you expose the body to conduct the exam.

D. have the crowd form a human barrier to protect you from oncoming traffic.

182. You arrive on the scene for a patient who is complaining of shortness of breath. As you enter, you note a large male patient weighing approximately 400 pounds sitting in a recliner. He is cyanotic and is on a nasal cannula at 2 lpm. You should immediately:

A. increase the oxygen flow to 6 lpm on the nasal cannula.

B. call for a backup crew to assist with lifting and moving the patient when ready to leave the scene.

C. place the patient on the floor and begin chest compressions.

D. ask the patient if he is able to walk down to the ambulance cot.

183. You are treating a patient who was struck in the head by a piece of machinery at a factory. Your partner tells you that the patient's airway is clear and he has a respiratory rate of 16/minute. You should immediately:

A. check for a radial pulse.

B. begin hyperventilating the patient by bag-valve-mask.

C. look at the chest for rise and fall and listen for air movement.

D. apply a nonrebreather at 15 lpm.

184. Your partner asks you to apply pressure to the anterior surface of the neck while he is ventilating in an attempt to reduce the risk of regurgitation and gastric distention. You will apply pressure to what anatomic structure?

A. glottic opening

B. epiglottis

C. thyroid cartilage

D. cricoid cartilage

185. Air flows from the nasopharynx immediately into the:

A. pharynx.

B. trachea.

C. larynx.

D. esophagus.

186. Which of the following statements about using an oropharyngeal airway is **true**?

A. It should never be removed once it is inserted.

B. It cannot be used while performing mouth-to-mask ventilation.

C. A head tilt-chin lift or jaw thrust maneuver must be maintained even with the airway in place.

D. A longer oropharyngeal airway can be used in cases of laryngeal swelling to facilitate airflow past the larynx.

187. You arrive on the scene of a construction site where you find a 26-year-old male patient who fell off a scaffold from about 25 feet. He is unresponsive, has blood in his mouth, and is breathing shallow at a rate of 24 per minute. You should immediately:

A. check for a radial and carotid pulse.

B. establish in-line spinal stabilization, suction the airway, and begin bag-valve-mask ventilation.

C. expose the patient and inspect for any open wounds to the chest.

D. establish in-line spinal stabilization, suction the airway, and apply a nonrebreather mask at 15 lpm.

188. When the intercostal muscles and diaphragm contract, the pressure in the chest becomes:
    A. negative.
    B. positive.
    C. equal to atmospheric pressure.
    D. greater than atmospheric pressure.

189. The major complication associated with flail segment is:
    A. pain on deep inhalation.
    B. hypoxia associated with an underlying pulmonary contusion.
    C. decreased breath sounds and tracheal deviation.
    D. stomach contents herniating into the chest cavity and impeding ventilation.

190. What part of the circulatory system acts as a reservoir for blood?
    A. arteries
    B. capillaries
    C. arterioles
    D. veins

191. What is the by-product of cellular metabolism when tissue perfusion is inadequate and the cells are hypoxic?
    A. lactic acid
    B. water and carbon dioxide
    C. carbon monoxide
    D. hydrogen chloride

192. What should the pressure be set at when suctioning the oropharynx of an adult patient?
    A. less than -120 mmHg
    B. -120 mmHg
    C. greater than -120 mmHg
    D. -80 to -100 mmHg

193. You are applying direct pressure to a large wound on the left forearm. The wound continues to bleed profusely even with the direct pressure. You should consider:
    A. applying a tourniquet.
    B. elevating the arm and apply pressure to the brachial artery.
    C. lowering the arm and apply cold packs to the wound.
    D. applying additional dressings and compressing the femoral artery.

194. When you arrive on the scene, the patient opens his eyes when you ask what happened. The patient is said to be:
    A. alert.
    B. responding to verbal stimuli.
    C. responding to painful stimuli.
    D. unresponsive.

195. Fractures not associated with major bleeding should be identified and managed during the:
    A. initial assessment.
    B. resuscitation phase.
    C. detailed physical exam.
    D. ongoing assessment.

196. Which of the following signs or symptoms would be an indication of an esophageal rupture?
    A. bowel sounds in the chest cavity
    B. jugular venous distention
    C. subcutaneous emphysema
    D. hemoptysis

197. Which of the following would **not** be considered a part of the history of the present illness (chief complaint)?
    A. medications
    B. onset
    C. severity
    D. duration

198. You are treating a 21-year-old female who was thrown from her horse. She is responding to painful stimuli with flexion of her arms. Her BP is 100/82 mmHg, heart rate is 126/minute, respirations of 34/minute and shallow. She has an obvious deformity and fracture to her left humerus. Prior to transport, you should:

    A. apply a nonrebreather mask, immobilize the humerus with a vacuum splint, and cover her with a blanket.

    B. begin bag-valve-mask ventilation, immobilize her to a backboard, immobilize the humerus to the backboard.

    C. immobilize her to a backboard, apply a nonrebreather mask, and splint the humerus with long boards and cravats.

    D. apply a cervical collar, apply a non-rebreather mask, splint the humerus with wire ladder splints.

199. The EMT's primary responsibility at the scene of motor vehicle crash is to:

    A. gain entry to the vehicle and provide emergency care to the patient.

    B. determine the best method to extricate the patient.

    C. instruct the extrication team on disentanglement of the patient.

    D. stay out of the vehicle until the patient is removed by the extrication team.

200. Which of the following statements about using lights and sirens to respond to an emergency is **true**?

    A. You have the right of way in all circumstances.

    B. You do not have to stop for any red lights or stop signs.

    C. You can pass a school bus but on the right side only.

    D. You must drive with due regard to others.

201. En route to the hospital following a motor vehicle crash the patient begins to complain of abdominal pain. Your next most appropriate action would be:

    A. stop the ambulance and take another blood pressure.

    B. apply the automated external defibrillator.

    C. reassess the abdomen by inspecting and palpating.

    D. auscultate for bowel sounds to determine if an intra-abdominal bleed exists.

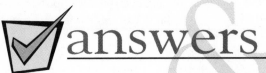

answers & rationales

1.

D. In the scene size-up, you identify potential environmental or situational hazards, secure the scene, determine MOI, locate patients, determine the number of patients, and assess the need for additional resources. *(1.6.2)*

2.

C. Using police assistance, if necessary, you should move the patient to your ambulance. The best way to deal with an environment that has become hostile is to get out of it. *(1.6.5)*

3.

D. The assessment of a medical patient is more commonly directed toward history gathering and a physical exam which tends to support the reported symptoms. Assessment of the trauma patient is directed toward identifying signs of injury. *(1.6.9)*

4.

A. The function of the vocal cords is to regulate the passage of air into the trachea and control the production of sound. *(1.6.12)*

5.

D. Simultaneously, air enters the nose and mouth and then moves into the pharynx where it enters the trachea via the larynx. *(1.6.13)*

6.

A. The function of turbinates is to warm and humidify air as it moves into the airway. *(1.6.14)*

7.

D. Air moves into the lungs when the alveolar pressure is lower than atmospheric pressure and moves out of the lungs when the alveolar pressure exceeds atmospheric pressure. *(1.6.21)*

8.

C. An injury to the diaphragm can impair its ability to contract normally. This reduces the size of the thoracic cavity, reducing ventilation. Some diaphragmatic injuries can result in the protrusion of abdominal contents into the thoracic cavity. *(1.6.23)*

9.

C. Esophageal intubation may be recognized by the absence of any resistance to ventilation, gastric distention, or the presence of breath sounds over the epigastrium. Increased airway resistance may be due to tension pneumothorax, occlusion of the airway, or intubation of the right main stem bronchus. *(1.6.24)*

10.

B. An increase in airway pressure would increase resistance to ventilation, making it more difficult to deflate the reservoir. Deflated reservoir bags may indicate an empty oxygen cylinder, a leak in the system, or a disconnected oxygen supply line. *(1.6.26)*

11.

B. Cervical spine injury, an intact gag reflex, and epiglottitis are relative contraindications to oral intubation. *(1.6.33)*

12.

B. Inadequate tourniquet pressure will only inhibit venous return and will not affect arterial flow, thus increasing the rate and volume of blood loss. Tourniquets should only be used as a last resort for hemorrhage control and, once applied, should not be released. A sphygmomanometer can be an effective tourniquet if it is inflated to 20 to 30 mmHg above the patient's systolic blood pressure. *(1.6.36)*

13.

C. It is important to fully expose your trauma patient during the assessment. Only through visualization, auscultation, palpation, and inspection can you identify potentially life-threatening. *(1.6.38)*

14.

C. For a 60-year-old male patient complaining of chest pain, it would be important to include information about his coronary bypass surgery last year. Pertinent past medical history should include information about preexisting medical problems, recent surgeries, medications, allergies, and the name of the patient's personal physician. *(1.6.45)*

15.

B. The definitive care phase of the patient care continuum includes the patient's admission to an appropriate receiving facility for surgical evaluation of traumatic injuries or management of an acute medical problem. *(1.6.47)*

16.

C. Manually stabilize the head and neck in a neutral position and apply the cervical collar. Then maintain cervical spine stabilization while log rolling the patient onto a long backboard. Strap the torso and legs securely to the board then secure the patient's head and neck. Secure the backboard to the cot. Immobilizing in this order improves control over the spine and reduces extraneous movement. *(1.6.50)*

17.

B. Continued evaluation, including serial measurement of vital signs will provide important information about a patient's condition. Vitals should be reassessed every 5 minutes in an unstable patient and every 15 minutes in a stable patient. During the ongoing assessment, you should also reassess the mental status, airway, ventilation, and circulatory status. Also, check all interventions and further assess any patient complaints. *(1.6.57)*

18.

A. Before CPR and suctioning are initiated, abdominal thrusts with blind finger sweeps must be continued in an attempt to alleviate the complete airway obstruction. For oxygenation of the patient's red blood cells to occur, a patent pathway for air movement must be secured to allow oxygen to enter the body. In this case, an obstructed airway is the highest priority. Chest thrusts are not indicated because they are not as effective as abdominal thrusts and are only performed on obese or pregnant patients. *(1.6.1)*

19.

B. Following an initial assessment, putting the patient in the ambulance is a priority based on the possibility of hypothermia. Since it is 2:00 A.M. and the patient is wet, the EMT-Intermediate must be alert to the likelihood of hypothermia and its potential effects on the patient. Removing the patient from the cold environment is a critical concern. *(1.6.4)*

20.

C. The division between upper and lower airway occurs at the level of the larynx. The upper airway structures are those found superior to the larynx while the lower airway begins at the level of the larynx. The larynx contains the vocal cords. *(1.6.11)*

21.

D. If the patient is groaning loudly, one must assume that the endotracheal tube has been misplaced in the esophagus. The vocal cords lie in the larynx and function to produce sound as passing air vibrates the cords. If an endotracheal tube is properly placed, air should not be vibrating the cords. In this case, one must deduce that the patient is able to produce sound because of the misplaced tube, so the tube placement must be checked immediately. *(1.6.12)*

22.

A. During inspiration, the diaphragm contracts, thereby increasing the volume of the lungs. As volume increases, pressure decreases below the pressure outside the body. Physical laws dictate that air will flow from an area of high concentration to one of low concentration. Therefore, air is drawn from outside the body into the lungs. *(1.6.13)*

23.

B. The visceral pleura immediately surrounds the external surface of the lung. The parietal pleura line the thoracic wall and the diaphragm. The alveoli comprise the bulk of the lung tissue itself. *(1.6.20)*

24.

C. The exchange of oxygen and carbon dioxide at the alveolar-capillary membrane is driven by differences in concentration. Gases typically flow from an area of higher concentration to that of a lower concentration in effort to achieve equilibrium. Oxygen molecules exist at a higher concentration in the alveoli than in the capillaries, therefore oxygen diffuses from the alveoli to the capillaries. The same can be said about how carbon dioxide moves from the capillaries to the alveoli. *(1.6.22)*

25.

D. This patient appears to be suffering from an open pneumothorax, which is compromising ventilatory status and creating a hypoxic state. Therefore your primary concern involves correcting this poor oxygenation state. An EMT-Intermediate should never open a chest wound to determine depth. Rather, the chest wound should be covered with an occlusive dressing to prevent the worsening of a pneumothorax. *(1.6.23)*

26.

A. Mouth-to-pocket mask ventilation provides the most reliable delivery of tidal volume during artificial ventilation. Because both hands are free to hold the mask to the face, a tight seal can be easily maintained. Also, the rescuer easily feels end inspiratory compliance as he or she blows into the pocket mask. The demand valve resuscitator and the bag-valve-mask do not maintain these properties in comparison to the pocket mask. A non-rebreathing mask does not deliver oxygen in terms of a tidal volume. *(1.6.25)*

27.

A. You would continue to ventilate at a rate of 12–20/minute. *(1.6.32)*

28.

A. Splinting this extremity would be the best way to control and prevent further hemorrhage. Splinting prevents the movement of sharp bone fragments that could lacerate other vessels and promulgate any bleeding. Also, the bones themselves contain vessels that must be stabilized so as to allow proper clotting mechanisms to take effect. The administration of oxygen is always indicated but does little for direct hemorrhage control. *(1.6.35)*

29.

C. A mini-neurological examination utilizing the mnemonic AVPU is a simple, objective way of quickly determining and conveying a patient's mental status. A = Alert, responds appropriately; V = responds to Verbal stimuli; P = responds to Painful stimuli; U = Unresponsive. *(1.6.37)*

30.

C. The Glasgow Coma Scale is a useful scoring system that can assist with monitoring neurologic status. Repeated values of the GCS can provide trends in mental status over a period of time. The parameters used for evaluation include eye, verbal, and motor response, not sensory. A number should not dictate the interventions an EMT-Intermediate must provide. Patient care is based upon an individual patient assessment/treatment process. *(1.6.44)*

31.

B. The EMT-Intermediate should consider obtaining at least one red-top blood tube. Red-top blood tubes do not contain any additives and many tests can be performed on the blood contained inside, for example, glucose levels, electrolytes, serum, etc. Although many hospitals routinely draw their own samples, prehospital blood is often utilized if the tubes are not expired, obtained with proper technique, and properly labeled. *(1.6.46)*

32.

B. Any time the EMT-Intermediate immobilizes an individual to a long board, the straps must be secured in the order of torso first, and head last. Straps are secured in this order to avoid further manipulation of the cervical spine as might happen if the head was secured initially and the torso moved during strapping. It is easiest to secure the legs after the torso. *(1.6.49)*

33.

C. Complete, accurate, and thorough documentation written at the time of patient refusal is always your best protection. "If it wasn't written down, it wasn't done," applies to every aspect of EMS from ambulance checklists to patient assessment and refusals. It is often hard to prove that verbal discussions took place and the present testimony of your partner may not accurately reflect the events that took place some time ago. Also, a standard refusal form without a written narrative is incomplete in that there is nothing to prove that any assessment was ever completed. *(1.6.56)*

34.

B. Your safety should be the first consideration. You should never enter a building that is not safe. When dealing with gas fumes or leaks, you should park your ambulance on the same level, or above and upwind from the hazardous material site. Hazardous materials experts will need to deal with the toxic substance and will be responsible for extricating the patients from the building. *(1.6.3)*

35.

C. You should keep your ambulance at a safe distance until the scene is safe. An injured EMT-Intermediate cannot render aid to the patient. Explain the situation to your dispatcher and have them notify the police for assistance. Take cover from the person with the weapon. *(1.6.5)*

36.

B. It is appropriate for you to transport the patient, initiate treatment, and meet your backup en route. An unconsciousness multiple system trauma patient fits the criteria for rapid transport. *(1.6.8)*

37.

C. Since the vocal cords are responsible for the production of sound and the larynx contains the vocal cords an injury to this structure could cause voice and airway dysfunction. Sounds could still be produced with injuries to the other structures listed. *(1.6.12)*

38.

B. Edema from any cause to the oropharynx is critical. The oropharynx serves to conduct air from both the nose and mouth into the larynx. An occlusion at any level of the upper airway may compromise ventilation and oxygenation. *(1.6.15)*

39.

C. The jaw thrust is the appropriate airway maneuver for the trauma patient because it allows neutral alignment of the cervical spine. The head tilt-chin lift requires hyperextension of the head, which is inappropriate for the trauma patient. *(1.6.16)*

40.

D. If the first attempt at ventilation is unsuccessful, the American Heart Association recommends repositioning the patient's head and trying another ventilation. Then abdominal thrusts, a finger sweep, and an attempt to ventilate, in that order, are appropriate. *(1.6.17)*

41.

C. When using a pocket mask, both hands can be utilized to maintain proper head tilt and a tight seal to the face while blowing through the protruding tube with your mouth. The bag-valve-mask requires one hand on the bag and the other on the mask, thus making it difficult to maintain a mask seal. Utilizing a second person would improve the dilemma, but was not an option in this scenario. Inserting an oropharyngeal airway only serves to secure the tongue and does nothing for the seal. Removal of the patient's dentures could worsen the situation by creating a void the bag-valve-mask has difficulty fitting. Finally, taping the mask is inappropriate. *(1.6.24)*

42.

C. Minimal bag resistance and rapid emptying is associated with a mask leak. During normal ventilations there should be moderate resistance. An airway obstruction creates significant resistance and a bag-valve-mask would not function correctly with a hole in the bag. *(1.6.26)*

43.

C. Abdominal distention can be a sign of too much pressure while ventilating, which causes air to be forced into the stomach. Abdominal distention can decrease the effectiveness of ventilations. Chest rise and fall, bilateral breath sounds, and decreased cyanosis are all signs of effective ventilation. *(1.6.27)*

44.

B. The patient would present as pale, cool, and clammy because of the body's compensatory mechanisms. The body shunts blood to the core organs in an effort to preserve them. *(1.6.29)*

45.

D. Leave the tourniquet in place and transport. Because the tourniquet was applied 2 hours ago, the EMT-Intermediate can assume that clots and acid have accumulated in the stagnant circulation. Any loosening or removal of the tourniquet could dislodge such clots and send the acidic blood into the systemic circulation. *(1.6.36)*

46.

C. Exposing the trauma patient is necessary to find life-threatening injuries. This should be limited only when the environment, bystanders, or the situation hinders exposure. Because of the weather, this patient should be exposed in the back of the ambulance. Make sure the patient is kept warm. *(1.6.39)*

47.

D. Priority would be given to the reassessment of the patient's distal pulse. When reassessing the patient, one must repeat the initial assessment, vital signs, focused assessment of the patient's complaint, and a check of all interventions. *(1.6.41)*

48.

D. Packaging includes all the actions necessary to prepare the patient for transportation. This includes emergency care procedures such as initiating airway control, ventilations, IVs, fracture stabilization, bandaging, and immobilization. *(1.6.48)*

49.

D. All patients should be secured to the cot before transfer to the ambulance. Many of the transport devices today only have three straps to secure the patient to the device. Patients who are secured to a backboard must also be secured to the cot. *(1.6.50)*

50.

C. Family wishes should be considered, however, the patient's condition can dictate which facility is most appropriate. When a patient's condition deteriorates, such as in this scenario, he or she should be transported to the closest appropriate facility for stabilization. Once stable, the patient can always be transferred to another hospital if the family wishes. *(1.6.53)*

51.

C. An assessment of the patient is necessary to identify and manage life threats and establish priorities of care. Transport decisions are made based on the assessment, but that is not the sole purpose of the assessment. Vital signs are only one component of the physical assessment and not its purpose. *(1.6.1)*

52.

B. Biological agents or germ-infested materials are some of the environmental dangers that an EMT-Intermediate would most likely face at the scene of a medical emergency. *(1.6.3)*

53.

B. Once you have ensured your safety, you have the responsibility to protect the patient from further injury using whatever protective equipment is necessary. *(1.6.6)*

54.

D. Vital signs are a part of the secondary assessment or focused history and physical exam. The initial assessment includes AVPU, airway, breathing, and circulation. *(1.6.10)*

55.

A. Once air enters the oral cavity, it travels through the oropharynx, passes the epiglottis, through the glottic opening, passes the vocal cords, then the cricoid cartilage which is the last structure before the trachea begins. *(1.6.13)*

56.

D. Mucus production is an effort to humidify incoming air, and remove dirt and pollens. As air passes through the nasal cavity, three important functions occur: air is filtered by "bouncing off" various structures—the conchae, septum, and pharyngeal wall, is warmed to 37∞C, and is humidified to within 2 to 3 percent of full saturation. *(1.6.14)*

57.

B. In laryngitis the vocal cords become inflamed, but this does not impede airflow to the lungs. There can be both congenital and peripheral causes for decreased ventilation. Some of the peripheral causes include: trauma, drowning, foreign bodies, burns, anaphylaxis, laryngospasm, hematomas, and bilateral vocal cord paralysis. Epiglottitis can lead to airway obstruction caused by laryngospasm. *(1.6.15)*

58.

A. Oxygen is diffused across the alveolar-capillary membrane into the red blood cell where it binds with hemoglobin. It is then delivered to the cells. Carbon dioxide is picked up from the cells and delivered back across the alveolar-capillary membrane where it is exhaled. *(1.6.22)*

59.

D. All of the choices can affect oxygen concentrations in the blood. However, pulmonary embolism decreases a portion of pulmonary circulation because of a clot, reducing blood flow to the alveoli and available oxygen in the blood. *(1.6.24)*

60.

C. Although all four ways listed are acceptable, mouth-to-mask ventilation provides the best tidal volume and is easiest to perform. The other methods, in preferential order, are: two-person bag-valve-mask; flow-restricted, oxygen-powered ventilation device; and one-person bag-valve-mask. *(1.6.25)*

61.

B. Gastric distention is an indicator of improper positioning of the head or overinflation of the lungs. If a patient is being ventilated adequately, which is every 5 seconds for an adult or every 3 seconds for the pediatric patient, the chest should rise and fall with each ventilation, skin color will improve, the heart rate will return to normal, and the pulse oximeter (SPO$_2$) reading will increase. Ventilations that are delivered too quickly will cause gastric distention. The adult ventilation should be delivered over a 1.5- to 2-second period and an infant and child over a 1- to 1.5-second period. *(1.6.27)*

62.

B. Suction should only be applied while slowly removing the catheter. Suctioning can be accomplished by using either a rigid, tonsil-tip catheter only as far as one can visualize; or using a flexible, soft suction catheter. Additionally, the soft suction catheter can be inserted into the endotracheal tube. Suction is usually set at greater than -120 mmHg for oral suctioning or less than -120 mmHg for endotracheal suction. *(1.6.34)*

63.

C. The AVPU scale is the acronym used for evaluating a patient's mental status in the initial assessment. AVPU stands for: A—Alert; V—responds to Verbal stimuli; P—responds to Painful stimuli; U—Unresponsive. *(1.6.37)*

64.

D. It is important to expose areas of the body that are pertinent to the patient's complaint or situation. In this instance, her leg should be exposed for evaluation and treatment, but not as part of the initial assessment. This will be conducted as part of the focused history and physical exam. *(1.6.39)*

65.

D. Proteinuria is related to the amount of protein excreted in the urine. This is checked by analyzing the urine and not the blood. *(1.6.46)*

66.

A. At the conclusion of your initial assessment, you should have ascertained that this patient is in need of immediate ventilatory support. Do not delay transport to initiate IV therapy or apply a cardiac monitor. These procedures can be done en route to the closest appropriate trauma facility. *(1.6.48)*

67.

B. The primary concern for this trauma patient is airway management. While the other injuries may also be considered life threats, failure to establish and maintain an airway will doom any other resuscitative interventions. Therefore, suction the oral cavity, and begin ventilation because of the high respiratory rate and poor tidal volume. *(1.6.1)*

68.

A. Auscultation of breath sounds would be performed after application of the cervical collar and palpation of the head and chest. *(1.6.2)*

69.

C. Scene safety is a primary concern on any call. Failure to actively notice hazards places you, your partner, the patient, and bystanders at risk. Upon identification of a hazard, you must immediately notify the proper services to handle the emergency prior to entering the scene. In this instance, notifying the fire department is the best course of action to prevent possible injuries to yourself and others. *(1.6.4)*

70.

B. During patient extrication, care must be taken to minimize the chance of additional injury. This typically includes covering the patient with a protective medium while the fire department removes the body panels. It is also beneficial to have an EMT-Intermediate in the auto with the patient to explain what is going on, since extrication can be a frightening experience. *(1.6.7)*

71.

A. Of particular concern in an unresponsive patient is airway patency. Unresponsive patients are often unable to keep their airway open and clear of secretions. In unresponsive patients, the tongue may become displaced posteriorly from hypotonicity of the mandibular muscles and occlude the airway at the level of the oropharynx. The nasopharynx is superior to the oropharynx, while the laryngopharynx (also called the hypopharynx) is inferior to the oropharynx, and contains the epiglottis. *(1.6.11)*

72.

D. The sense of smell is achieved by a group of specialized olfactory cells located in the superior nasopharynx. The bony projections in the nasal cavity (called conchae or turbinates) cause the inspired air to become very turbulent. This allows any foreign material in the inspired air to become trapped on the mucosal lining. Since the lining is also vascular, it will impart moisture and allow for temperature modification. *(1.6.14)*

73.

A. The oropharyngeal airway is an adjunct to establishing a patent airway. Manual maneuvers must be maintained to ensure the airway is open and clear. *(1.6.16)*

74.

B. A simple closed pneumothorax occurs when air enters the pleural space between the visceral and parietal pleura. This causes a loss of negative intrapleural pressure causing the lung to partially collapse. *(1.6.23)*

75.

C. Trying to maintain an adequate seal of the mask while performing mouth-to-mask ventilations is one of the most common causes of difficulty. To perform this skill effectively, the EMT-Intermediate should be positioned behind the patient with his or her thumbs along each side of the mask; using the palms to push downward helps ensure a good seal. The index, middle, and ring fingers should then be placed on the mandible to lift and displace the mandible anteriorly. *(1.6.25)*

76.

D. Positive pressure ventilation is indicated whenever there is inadequate tidal volume or inadequate rate. While the normal minute volume is a function of respiratory rate and depth, if the depth is inadequate, it does not matter what the rate is. While a low SpO_2 reading and cyanosis both indicate poor oxygenation, they do not directly reflect respiratory tidal volume or rate and would warrant further evaluation. *(1.6.26)*

77.

A. The heart has the unique ability to initiate its own impulse causing depolarization. That ability is known as automaticity. The cells primary role is to initiate the depolarization wave resulting in organized contraction of the heart. Excitability is the ability of a cell to respond to an impulse, conductivity refers to the transmission of electrical impulses from cell to cell, and contractility refers to the actual muscular contraction of myocardial cells. *(1.6.28)*

78.

A. The femoral artery, by nature of carrying a large amount of blood under high pressure, is responsible for the profuse and spurting hemorrhage. Veins bleed continuously with a steady flow. The tibial and iliac arteries are not located in the upper thigh. *(1.6.35)*

79.

D. Paradoxical movement of the right thorax would be found during inspection. Inspection allows the EMT-

Intermediate to identify external signs of trauma/illness. Auscultation is necessary to discern bilateral wheezing, hyperresonance is a function of percussion, and crepitus is found during palpation. *(1.6.38)*

80.

A. Hypotension with bradycardia, differences in skin temperature and moisture, and a bounding pulse are characteristic of vasogenic shock secondary to spinal cord injury. The injury causes an interruption in the sympathetic nerve transmission, therefore, there is not a reflexive increase in the heart rate from the hypotension, and the interruption also results in compensatory changes above the level of injury and none below. Hypovolemic shock presents with hypotension, tachycardia, and diaphoresis. *(1.6.40)*

81.

B. Management of non–life threatening injuries is completed while en route to the hospital. Any life-threatening injury should be managed during the initial assessment and rapid trauma assessment. *(1.6.47)*

82.

A. After fully immobilizing a patient to a long backboard, the motor, sensory, and perfusion (MSP) status should be assessed in each extremity. *(1.6.49)*

83.

D. An open wound to the thorax is considered an immediate life-threatening injury that must be managed during the initial assessment or rapid trauma assessment. *(1.6.52)*

84.

C. The sequence is based on potential "threats to life." The airway is managed first, followed by breathing, then circulation. *(1.6.1)*

85.

B. A cold home is not a hazard that you are concerned with because of your short on-scene exposure. How-

ever, the cold home could provide important scene size-up clues as to the potential for hypothermia. *(1.6.4)*

86.

B. Delay entry into a hostile scene until arrival of law enforcement personnel. While an additional EMS unit may be needed, law enforcement is responsible for controlling a hostile scene. Numerous hazards can result in injury or death to the EMT-Intermediate. Think before taking a particular action and always assume the worse. Additional sources of hazards to the EMT-Intermediate include unstable surfaces, ice, and crowds. *(1.6.5)*

87.

C. Crowd control is primarily a law enforcement function. However, sometimes this may be provided by EMS until arrival of law enforcement. The use of EMT-Intermediates is acceptable only if enough resources are available. *(1.6.7)*

88.

D. The three common resources requested at emergency scenes include law enforcement, fire and rescue services, and electric utilities. The coroner's investigator may be frequently called but he/she should not be needed to enter the scene or begin patient care. *(1.6.8)*

89.

C. All items are correctly paired. The best answer is the incomplete answer. Obstetrics refers to pregnancy or childbirth. Gynecology is anything having to do with the female reproductive system. *(1.6.9)*

90.

D. The first item to evaluate in the initial assessment is the general impression. During the general impression you look for major life threats and determine the age and gender of the patient. *(1.6.10)*

91.

D. The purpose of the initial assessment is to quickly determine immediate life threats that may be present. Once discovered, these threats to life need to be managed immediately. *(1.6.10)*

92.

B. The pharynx is divided into three regions. The superior region is known as the nasopharynx and is located directly posterior to the nasal opening. The middle region is called the oropharynx and is posterior to the mouth. The inferior region of the pharynx is called the laryngopharynx or the hypopharynx. *(1.6.11)*

93.

C. The use of the jaw thrust maneuver maintains the head in a neutral position while moving the jaw forward. This displaces the tongue off the posterior oropharynx and opens the airway. Because the head is maintained in a neutral position, it is the airway method of choice for a trauma patient with a suspected spinal injury. *(1.6.16)*

94.

B. The patient has a partial airway obstruction. He is moving enough air to produce a cough so he should be encouraged to continue to cough. Watch the patient carefully for signs of inadequate breathing, such as a weak, ineffective cough, high-pitched wheezing during inhalation, increased difficulty in breathing, or the development of cyanosis. If any of these are present, treat this patient as if he had a complete airway obstruction. Deliver repeated abdominal thrusts until the patient loses consciousness or the obstruction is removed. If you are able to intubate, perform a laryngoscopy and remove the obstruction with the Magill forceps. *(1.6.17)*

95.

C. The jaw thrust is the only procedure listed that maintains the head in a neutral position. In the suspected spine injured patient, the spine must not be flexed, extended, or moved laterally. *(1.6.19)*

96.

C. The point at which the trachea divides into the right and left main stem bronchus is called the carina. The alveolar duct is the terminal portion of the respiratory tract just before it enters the alveoli. The cricoid is the most inferior portion of the larynx. *(1.6.20)*

97.

A. The connective tissue that covers the lungs is called the pleura. The pleura is a single membrane that doubles over itself to form what seems to be a double membrane. The outermost layer of the pleura is the parietal pleura. Next is a potential space called the pleural space and the innermost layer attached to the lung tissue is the visceral pleura. *(1.6.20)*

98.

D. The process of inhalation begins with the contraction of the diaphragm and the intercostal muscles. The diaphragm moves downward as the ribs move upward. This increases the total volume of air that can be contained within the thoracic cavity. This rapid change in volume creates a negative pressure in relationship to outside air pressure. As a result, air moves into the chest cavity to equalize this imbalance. *(1.6.21)*

99.

B. The process of exhalation is a passive process. Relaxation of the contracted diaphragm and intercostal muscles are the only actions required. The diaphragm moves upwards and the ribs move down. This action reduces the volume within the thoracic cavity. The air pressure is greater within the thoracic cavity than the atmospheric air. The air moves out of the thoracic cavity. *(1.6.21)*

100.

A. Carbon dioxide and oxygen move across the alveolar-capillary membrane in a process called diffusion. Diffusion is the movement of gases from an area of greater concentration to an area of lesser concentration. Oxygen moves from the alveoli to the capillary and carbon dioxide moves from the capillary to the alveoli. *(1.6.22)*

101.

A. The epicardium is the outermost layer of myocardial tissue. The other layers include the pericardial sac, the myocardium or middle layer containing muscle, and the endocardium or innermost layer. *(1.6.28)*

102.

A. The earliest detectable change that occurs with diminished blood volume is an increased heart rate. Increased cardiac stroke volume is difficult to detect clinically. Peripheral vasoconstriction will occur causing the skin to become pale, cool, and clammy. *(1.6.29)*

103.

D. If the radial pulse is absent because of poor perfusion, it is likely that the donsalis pedis and posterior tibial pulses would also be absent. The carotid and brachial arteries may still be perfused. It takes less blood pressure to perfuse the carotid, femoral, and brachial pulses as compared to a greater pressure to perfuse the posterior tibial and dorsalis pedis arteries. The apical pulse will be felt with any contraction of the heart. *(1.6.31)*

104.

D. When you are ventilating a patient with an esophageal obturator airway (EOA), you must maintain a tight mask seal. Any leak that occurs will diminish the volume of air delivered. The most common complication associated with the EOA is a poor mask seal leading to ineffective ventilation. *(1.6.32)*

105.

C. After tube placement, auscultate over the epigastric region and then over the right and left apex of the lungs. No gurgling sounds should be heard while auscultating over the stomach during ventilation. Note the equality of right and left breath sounds and watch for the chest to rise and fall. Air escaping from the nose and mouth is a sign of improper inflation or a leak in the cuff. The pulse oximeter is not used to check for proper tube placement because the reading may not be available in the patient and is delayed in many. *(1.6.33)*

106.

C. The suction catheter must initially be inserted into the endotracheal tube without suction applied. Measuring from the lips, then to the ear, and then to the nipple line places the suction catheter at about the level of the carina. Suction is applied and the catheter is removed with a twisting motion. Suction should not exceed 15 seconds. *(1.6.23)*

107.

D. The statement that best describes shock is inadequate delivery of oxygen to cells and inadequate elimination of CO_2 and other waste by-products. *(1.6.40)*

108.

A. The unstable patient should be reassessed every 5 minutes. The stable patient should be reassessed every 15 minutes. *(1.6.41)*

109.

B. Subcutaneous emphysema is a collection of air trapped under the skin. It is a sign of trauma to the airway, respiratory tract, lungs, or esophagus. Observe the patient closely for signs of a developing pneumothorax, tension pneumothorax, or hemothorax. A pericardial tamponade is a collection of fluid in the pericardium. A tension pneumothorax is a condition resulting from collection of air in the pleural space. A hematoma is a collection of blood under the skin. *(1.4.43)*

110.

D. The revised trauma score evaluates the respiratory rate, systolic blood pressure, and the Glasgow Coma Scale score. The respiratory rate and systolic blood pressure are assigned a numerical value based upon pre-established criteria. The Glasgow Coma Scale is performed and assigned a point value based upon a fixed scale. These two values are then added together to determine the patient's total trauma score. The trauma score is valuable to receiving hospitals for categorization and reassessment purposes. *(1.6.44)*

111.

C. Determining the patient's father's medical history is not considered a necessity during initial history taking. A SAMPLE history should be obtained and includes S = signs and symptoms, A = allergies, M = medications, P = past medical history, L = last oral intake, E = events prior to illness. Radiation of pain is an important component of the history of the present illness. *(1.6.45)*

112.

A. HIV testing is not a routine reason for the prehospital collection of blood samples. Blood glucose, CBC, and type and cross-match are common lab tests performed. *(1.6.46)*

113.

A. The ongoing assessment is performed to detect changes in patient condition, assess additional patient complaints, and to evaluate the treatment provided. The reassessment of patients should be performed every 5 minutes in the unstable patient and every 15 minutes in the stable patient. An ongoing assessment must be performed on a routine basis on all patients, regardless of time or patient condition. *(1.6.52)*

114.

C. The most important factor to determine the destination medical facility depends primarily upon which facility is best able to manage the patient. The transport of patients to specialized care centers will improve patient outcomes. Thus, the patient condition is a primary consideration. For the stable patient, the decision should be a joint determination reached between the patient and the EMT-Intermediate. *(1.6.53)*

115.

B. Patient care is frequently compromised when using the lights and siren. Additional stress is placed on the patient, the EMT-Intermediate, and the driver. Higher accident rates are associated with the use of lights and siren, not lower rates. Drive professionally and use lights and siren only when necessary. *(1.6.54)*

116.

C. Question the order by "echoing" the orders back to the medical control physician. Medical control may have misunderstood your description of the patient condition or history. Echoing the orders allows the physician to hear and correct a potentially inappropriate order. *(1.6.55)*

117.

A. During the ongoing assessment, the initial assessment of mental status, airway, breathing, and circulation is always repeated. The vital signs are also reassessed and a focused physical exam is performed if there are additional complaints. *(1.6.57)*

118.

A. The process of ensuring scene safety begins well before you arrive on the scene. Dispatch information may alert you to many hazards such as fallen wires, chemical hazards, potentially harmful diseases, and violent settings. *(1.6.2)*

119.

A. It is best to stage your vehicle and not approach the vehicle to avoid scene hazards. Wait for personnel that are specially trained to manage downed wires. *Never* attempt to remove any wires unless you have been specially trained. *(1.6.3)*

120.

C. If for any reason the scene turns hazardous, immediately remove yourself from the scene and return only when you are sure that it is safe. Always protect yourself and your partner first. Usually you cannot reason with a hostile crowd. Furthermore, asserting authority on a hostile scene will usually only exacerbate the situation. *(1.6.5)*

121.

D. There will be little time to go back to the vehicle for protective gear. You should have eye protection and gloves on before you exit your vehicle. An exposure can happen quickly. If you wait until you are at the patient's side before you have body substance isolation (BSI), the public may perceive this as not being prepared or not wanting to touch the patient. In addition, it delays patient care. *(1.6.6)*

122.

C. You accomplish two objectives by having the onlookers hold the unfolded sheet. You protect the patient's dignity while giving the bystanders a task to do. *(1.6.7)*

123.

B. If you determine that the number of patients exceeds your available resources, first get more help on the way by implementing the multiple casualty plan. The number of critically injured is not as important as requesting additional resources. Quickly treating life threats will come in the triage phase of the multiple casualty incident plan. Finally, making patient contact prior to calling for additional resources will cause you to become focused on the patient's needs and not the needs of the entire situation. *(1.6.8a)*

124.

A. If you are not trained for this special situation you should immediately call for a specialty trained swift water rescue team. You are taking an unnecessary risk by trying to rescue the patient without the proper training in swift water rescue. The bystanders may be swept down river and require rescuing. Even the strongest person cannot hold onto a rope for very long in a swift current. *(1.6.8b)*

125.

C. Your first impression is based on several things. The dispatcher's information, scene size-up, and bystander's remarks should lead you to categorize this patient as medical. As you gather more information and complete an assessment, you may need to recategorize the patient. *(1.6.9)*

126.

A. The mucous membrane has a rich blood supply which immediately warms, humidifies, and filters the inspired air. Inferior turbinate and superior conchae are bony projections that cause turbulent airflow which help to deposit airborne particles on the mucous membrane. External nares help to filter the air; however, they do not warm or humidify. *(1.6.14)*

127.

D. Stridor is associated with a life-threatening upper airway obstruction and can be caused by a foreign body, severe swelling, or a metabolic process. Presence of fluids in the upper airway will present with gurgling sounds. Constriction of the bronchioles present with wheezing. *(1.6.15)*

128.

B. Direct laryngoscopy is the visualization of the vocal cords and glottic opening using a laryngoscope. The Magill forceps can be used for foreign body removal but only in conjunction with direct visualization. Back blows should not be performed on an adult. This may cause further obstruction of the airway. Finger sweeps are not performed in conjunction with the Magill forceps. The oropharyngeal airway may push the obstruction further into the airway. *(1.6.17)*

129.

C. If the patient begins to cough or gag you must quickly remove the oropharyngeal airway or the patient may vomit and aspirate. Turning the patient to the side will not prevent the patient from vomiting, however, this position may decrease the chance of aspiration. Be prepared to use suction, but remove the airway first. Reassuring the patient will not reduce the gag reflex and stimulations that may cause vomiting and aspiration. *(1.6.18a)*

130.

C. Use only water-soluble lubricants with the airway. Petroleum products may cause further injury to the nasal mucosa and tissue and damage the nasopharyngeal airway. Insert the airway with the bevel towards the septum then straight back into the nasopharynx. The airway is measured from the tip of the nose to the tip of the earlobe. *(1.6.18b)*

131.

D. The jaw-thrust maneuver is used to open the airway in patients with suspected spine trauma. Sonorous sounds indicate the tongue is partially occluding the airway. Thus, using the jaw thrust and an oropharyngeal airway, the airway should be opened adequately. This technique does not require hyperextension of the head to open the airway. The Sellick's maneuver describes the pressure applied to the cricoid cartilage to close off the esophagus and improve the view of the vocal cords during intubation. *(1.6.19a)*

132.

A. The skin above the site of spine injury becomes pale, cool, and clammy; whereas the skin below the site becomes warm and dry. *(1.6.19b)*

133.

D. Gas exchange occurs in the alveoli of the lungs. The lungs are covered with connective tissue called the pleura. The alveolar ducts and terminal bronchioles serve as a primary conduit and not as exchange components. *(1.6.20)*

134.

C. The bag-valve-mask is more difficult to use than a pocket mask, therefore, one-person ventilation is achieved better with the pocket-mask. Two EMTs are recommended to maintain a good mask seal and deliver a greater tidal volume. The pocket mask can deliver a greater tidal volume than the bag-valve-mask. Nearly 100 percent concentration of oxygen can be delivered by the bag-valve-mask when used with supplemental high flow oxygen, as well as a reservoir bag or tubing. *(1.6.26)*

135.

D. A pop-off valve that continues to vent air may not allow sufficient volumes to be delivered. A heart rate that returns to normal is a sign of adequate ventilations. Good chest rise indicates an adequate tidal volume, which indicates adequate ventilation. Dry, warm, and pink skin are good indications of adequate ventilation. *(1.6.27)*

136.

D. When sufficient oxygen is present (aerobic metabolism) and perfusion is adequate, pyruvic acid breaks down into carbon dioxide, water, and energy. This is known as the Kreb's cycle. The others may result from decreased perfusion and lead to cellular death which may lead to death of the organism. *(1.6.29)*

137.

A. Coronary artery disease is the leading cause of cardiac arrest and sudden death (death that occurs within one hour of the onset of symptoms). The other answers are all causes of cardiac arrest, however, they do not occur more frequently than death from coronary artery disease. *(1.6.30)*

138.

A. Delayed capillary refill is not a reliable indicator of inadequate perfusion in the adult patient. Environmental factors, gender, and medications can alter capillary refill in the adult. Capillary refill is a quick method to check peripheral perfusion in young children. Cool skin does not alone indicate poor perfusion. The pupil will dilate and respond sluggishly to light in poor perfusion states. *(1.6.31)*

139.

D. The next immediate action in this patient is to establish an airway followed by management of the inadequate ventilation status. A pulse will be assessed after establishing a patent airway and adequate ventilations. Vitals will be assessed after the initial assessment and during the rapid trauma assessment. *(1.6.32)*

140.

D. To properly assess a trauma patient, you must completely expose the body. Non–life-threatening injuries are treated after the rapid trauma assessment is complete. *(1.6.38)*

141.

A. When the patient is in a cold environment, it may be dangerous to expose the patient until transfer to the ambulance. If a crowd is present, protect the dignity of the patient by covering him or her with a sheet. *(1.6.39)*

142.

D. The most reliable indicator of a head injury is deteriorating mental status. *(1.6.41)*

143.

A. Application of a cervical spinal immobilization collar is not done during the detailed physical exam. It is applied during the rapid trauma assessment. *(1.6.42)*

144.

B. Subcutaneous emphysema is air trapped under the skin. It is a good indicator of a significant chest injury. The air that is trapped may come from a leak in the trachea, bronchus, lungs, or the esophagus. A flail segment may cause the paradoxical movement and is a serious chest injury. Suprasternal notch retraction is a serious sign that the patient is having a difficult time breathing and needs immediate management. *(1.6.43)*

145.

B. The respiratory rate is not evaluated when using the Glasgow Coma Score. The GCS is a system used to monitor neurologic status. The trauma score incorporates the evaluation of the respiratory rate and effort in addition to perfusion status. *(1.6.44)*

146.

D. The portable ambulance cot has a load capacity of up to 350 pounds. However, it is not recommended for that much weight. You should try to use at least four other rescuers. Canvas cots offer no support for spinal injuries and should be used only in conjunction with a long backboard. Loading the wheeled ambulance cot first will not permit the room needed to safely load the portable cot. *(1.6.50)*

147.

C. The primary concern at the scene is safety. An unstable vehicle should not be entered until it is made safe. *(1.6.51)*

148.

D. You should perform a focused assessment of the complaint. Oxygen or nitroglycerin will not relieve the pain. Performing a detailed physical exam is unnecessary. *(1.6.52)*

149.

C. A Glasgow Coma Score of less than 9 indicates a significant neurologic deficit. A humerus fracture with no major bleeding is not a great concern. The frontal collision is a mechanism that needs to be correlated with clinical signs and symptoms to determine the priority status of a patient. *(1.6.53)*

150.

C. When you provide a complete report, care can be continued without interruption. Medical care consists of events that require consistency to enhance patient care. *(1.6.55)*

151.

A. Your written report will not prevent you from being sued in court, however, a well-written report is your best defense in a court of law. You should use a standardized format. All run reports do become a permanent part of the patient's medical record. Many physicians, nurses, and other health care providers rely on the run report to convey the complete picture of the event. *(1.6.56)*

152.

B. Assessment and treatment priorities of the initial assessment, threats to the airway, breathing, and circulation are treated immediately upon identification. It is necessary to take in-line spinal immobilization, clear the airway, and then manage the insufficient ventilating status. *(1.6.1)*

153.

C. The patient is alert and talking, therefore the airway is patent and the breathing is adequate. Your next immediate action is to administer oxygen and assess circulation. *(1.6.7)*

154.

B. Managing the airway on an unresponsive patient may be challenging, especially if the gag reflex is still intact. If a manual technique fails in the patient, reposition the airway again before going to a mechanical airway. *(1.6.18)*

155.

B. There are numerous ways the EMT-I can deliver artificial ventilations to a patient. Mouth-to-mask ventilation has been shown to provide a greater tidal volume during ventilations. *(1.6.25)*

156.

D. Scene safety is the first priority on any call. It takes precedence over all other assessments or interventions. *(1.6.31)*

157.

D. The initial assessment is performed to identify and manage life-threats to the airway, breathing, and circulation. Hypotension will be identified by a blood pressure, which is not taken until the rapid assessment or focused physical exam. *(1.6.42)*

158.

C. During the process of immobilization you must be careful to not aggravate any existing injuries. Once on the backboard immobilize the torso of the body first and then head. Strapping in this order allows the rescuer to protect the head and neck from pivoting. *(1.6.49)*

159.

A. In the responsive medical patient, the most reliable information is gained from the patient in the history. The physical exam is then guided by the complaint of the patient. Therefore, you obtain a SAMPLE history followed by a focused physical exam and then obtain a set of baseline vital signs. *(1.6.9)*

160.

B. The EMT-I should provide treatment based on his or her protocol given the patient's chief complaint. The wishes of others on scene (physicians, family, bystanders, or partners) may be considered, but if it causes deviation from your protocol you must first contact medical control to get approval. *(1.6.55)*

161.

C. During the management of a patient with a partially occluded airway, the EMT-I should progress in a systematic fashion, employing those techniques which are most likely to work first and the most quickly. As such, if the patient displays sonorous respirations, the EMT-I should first use manual airway techniques, followed by simple and then advanced mechanical techniques to open the airway. *(1.6.16)*

162.

C. Adequate ventilations are best confirmed by equal breath sounds in all lung fields. Although the EMT-I should note diminishing cyanosis as the patient is oxygenated, this will take longer to become apparent. The absence of gastric sounds only indicates the ET tube is not in the esophagus. Adequate ventilation should produce CO_2 that can be detected by an end-tidal CO_2 monitor. *(1.6.33)*

163.

D. Oxygen and carbon dioxide diffuse across the alveoli, moving from higher to lower concentrations. As such, oxygen leaves the alveoli and diffuses into the capillary where it eventually attaches to hemoglobin on red blood cells. Carbon dioxide travels in the opposite direction. It leaves the capillary, enters the alveoli, and is expelled during exhalation. *(1.6.22)*

164.

D. Whenever the body is not meeting the metabolic demands, shock (or hypoperfusion) will result. Obstructive shock results from a tension pneumothorax, pulmonary embolism, and pericardial tamponade. *(1.6.40)*

165.

D. A run report is the most important document you will complete following any emergency call. It can be used for quality improvement purposes, it can become a part of billing, it may be reviewed for legal concerns, and it is needed to assure appropriate treatment is rendered after delivering the patient to the emergency department. The prehospital care report becomes a part of the patient's permanent record. *(1.6.56)*

166.

A. Generally, you should obtain a venous blood sample whenever an IV is initiated in the prehospital environment. You should always consider drawing blood on a patient suspected of being hypoglycemic, especially prior to the administration of 50 percent dextrose. A patient with an altered mental status and bizarre behavior may potentially be hypoglycemic. *(1.6.46)*

167.

C. There is no best way around this situation. A car on fire is not a safe scene by any means. Until it is possible to attempt extrication, you need to offer some type of protection. Since trying to outfit the patient in turnout gear would be nearly impossible, attempt to cover him or her with some flame retardant material such as a blanket. *(1.6.6)*

168.

A. A flail segment diminishes the bellows action of the chest. This does not allow that portion of the underlying lung to expand with the rest of the thorax. This diminishes the tidal volume and will result in hypoxemia and hypercapnia. A flail segment does not impact the airway, nor guarantee that a hemo- or pneumothorax is present. Diaphragm paralysis is not a result of fractured ribs. *(1.6.23)*

169.

C. Sound is produced when air that is exiting the trachea causes the vocal cords to vibrate. Speech is produced by a combination of vocal cord vibration and changes in the pharynx due to muscular contraction. The trachea cannot really change diameter because of cartilaginous support. *(1.6.12)*

170.

B. Realistically, the provision of cardiopulmonary resuscitation (CPR) is to prolong the viability of the patient until defibrillation and advanced life support providers can provide additional drug therapy and airway skills. CPR alone does not treat the underlying cause of arrest, and rarely (if ever) restores normal cardiac activity. *(1.6.30)*

171.

B. The purpose of the detailed physical exam is to identify and treat non–life-threatening injuries. Evisceration, open femur fracture, and the knife wound are all considered life-threatening injuries that should be detected and treated in the initial assessment phase. *(1.6.47)*

172.

D. In the management of a patient with an active hemorrhage, the progression of management should be direct pressure, elevation, application of cold, pressure point, tourniquet. *(1.6.36)*

173.

C. Two units following each other when running lights and siren can be problematic because motorists usually anticipate only one unit at a time. As such, when one passes the motorists typically resume normal traffic. This could cause problems for the second responding unit. *(1.6.54)*

174.

C. After manual techniques have failed to remove a foreign body airway obstruction, the next best thing is to perform a laryngoscopy and retrieve the obstruction with Magill forceps. Initiating transport will do nothing for the airway obstruction, and waiting until the patient arrests only makes the situation worse. Finally, back blows are not recommended as appropriate treatment for adults. *(1.6.17)*

175.

B. During intubation, it is important that you take appropriate BSI precautions to protect yourself from splashes or droplets. Since it is not uncommon for the patient to gag or cough during the skill, the bare minimum protection you would want is gloves for your hands, eye protection, and a mask for your mouth. A gown is usually not warranted unless there is a large amount of blood or other body fluids that may be splashed on you. *(1.6.3)*

176.

B. The appropriate term to use when removing a patient from their initial location is known as extrication. Since using appropriate terminology is imperative when interfacing with other health care providers and rescue personnel, you should use the correct term whenever possible. The other terms may be similar or understandable but they still do not represent the most correct term. *(1.6.51)*

177.

A. When a person is intubated, the vocal cords are spread by the endotracheal tube. This means that no air will pass over the cords during exhalation and as such, no sound can be produced. A facemask is irrelevant because one is not used once the patient is successfully intubated. And finally, PPV has no bearing on whether or not the vocal cords contract or not. *(1.6.12)*

178.

D. Your first priority at any scene is to establish scene safety. If the scene is not safe, you must either make it safe or retreat until another agency, such as law enforcement or the fire service, can make it safe for you. *(1.6.2)*

179.

A. Determining if the perpetrator is still on the scene is a scene safety issue, which is always a priority. If the perpetrator is still on the scene, it is considered a scene safety hazard. You would not enter the scene until it is safe. *(1.6.4)*

180.

B. Body substance isolation is considered a priority in your scene size-up. A patient who is ill, has a fever, and is coughing up blood-tinged sputum, may have tuberculosis or another respiratory illness. It is necessary to use gloves, eye protection, and a high efficiency particulate air (HEPA) respirator to protect you from the potential transmission of the TB bacteria or other infectious material. *(1.6.6)*

181.

C. Even when the scene is very hectic and uncontrolled, it is necessary to always protect the patient's modesty. Once you have exposed the trauma patient and inspected for injuries, cover the patient with a sheet or blanket to protect him or her. This may be enough to drastically reduce the patient's anxiety. *(1.6.7)*

182.

B. During your scene size-up, you are also looking for personal hazards that may cause injury to you or your partner. When you note an extremely large patient that you feel you and your partner cannot safely lift or move, you should immediately call for assistance. By calling for a backup during the scene size-up, you may reduce the time you are on the scene by having extra personnel available as soon as the patient is ready to be moved. *(1.6.8)*

183.

C. In order to insure that the breathing is adequate, you must assess both rate and tidal volume. In this scenario, the rate was assessed, however, the quality of breathing was not. The patient could be breathing 16/minute with a minimal tidal volume in which the patient would need to be ventilated. A respiratory rate alone does not establish adequate or inadequate breathing. *(1.6.10)*

184.

D. The cricoid cartilage is the circumferential ring that is compressed while performing cricoid pressure, also known as Sellick's maneuver. The cricoid ring is the big bulky cartilage immediately inferior (below) the thyroid cartilage (Adam's apple). Between the cricoid and thyroid cartilage is the cricothyroid membrane. *(1.6.11)*

185.

A. The air flows from the nasopharynx into the pharynx. From there the air moves into the hypopharynx, where the opening to the larynx (glottic opening) and esophagus are found. *(1.6.13)*

186.

C. Oropharyngeal or nasopharyngeal airways are considered airway adjuncts. Even with either of these airways in place, you must still maintain a manual maneuver, such as a head tilt-chin lift or jaw thrust. *(1.6.18)*

187.

B. According to your priority of care, you should establish in-line spinal stabilization, suction the airway, and begin bag-valve-mask ventilation. The patient's breathing is shallow indicating the need to ventilate. Once you have cleared the airway and begun ventilation, you then move on to check the pulse and skin. *(1.6.19)*

188.

A. When the intercostal muscles and diaphragm contract, the size of the thorax increases making the pressure inside negative. Because the intrathoracic pressure is lower than atmospheric pressure, air flows into the lungs resulting in inhalation. *(1.6.21)*

189.

B. The major problem associated with a flail segment are the underlying lung injury (pulmonary contusion) and the hypoxia associated with it. You can easily correct the pressure disturbance caused by an ineffective bellow action of the chest by simply ventilating the patient. However, it is the disturbance in gas exchange and oxygenation at the alveolar level from tissue destruction and bleeding in the lung tissue that is not easily corrected. *(1.6.24)*

190.

D. The venous system is known as the reservoir or capacitance system. It houses the majority of blood. Whether the arterial or venous vessels are damaged, the venous volume decreases. This decrease in preload of the heart reduces the cardiac output, perfusion, and eventually the blood pressure. *(1.6.28)*

191.

A. When cells do not receive an adequate amount of oxygen, they change from aerobic (with oxygen) to anaerobic (without oxygen) metabolism. The by-product of aerobic metabolism is water and carbon dioxide, whereas the by-product of anaerobic metabolism is lactic acid. *(1.6.30)*

192.

C. When suctioning the oropharynx of an adult patient, set the suction to exceed –120 mmHg of pressure. When performing enotracheal suctioning, the pressure is set at –80 to –120 mmHg. *(1.6.34)*

193.

B. If direct pressure fails to control the bleeding, your next method for bleeding control is pressure points. In this scenario, the brachial artery will be compressed to reduce the blood flow to the lower forearm while direct pressure is maintained. The tourniquet is a last resort if all other bleeding control measures fail. *(1.6.35)*

194.

B. The patient is responding to verbal stimuli. If he had his eyes open upon your arrival, he would be considered alert. If he opened his eyes to a pinch or other noxious stimuli, he would be responsive to painful stimuli. *(1.6.37)*

195.

C. Fracture management is done during the detailed physical exam. Fractures are not considered life-threatening injuries unless they are associated with major bleeding. One exception is a femur fracture because a patient can lose up to two liters of blood around each femur. *(1.6.42)*

196.

C. Subcutaneous emphysema, air trapped under the skin, is a sign of an air leak in the thorax or neck. Air may come from the trachea, bronchi, bronchioles, alveoli, or esophagus. *(1.6.43)*

197.

A. Medications are not considered part of the history of the present illness. The OPQRST mnemonic is used to gather information about the chief complaint. Medications are part of the SAMPLE history. *(1.6.45)*

198.

B. You would perform bag-valve-mask ventilation due to the inadequate volume of respiration, immobilize the patient to the backboard because of suspicion of a spinal injury related to the mechanism of injury, and simply strap the humerus to the backboard as a method of immobilization. This patient is considered a priority patient. Taking the time to immobilize the humerus fracture at the scene is not appropriate unless it will not lengthen the scene time. The backboard will serve as a splint until further immobilization can be performed en route. *(1.6.48)*

199.

A. An EMT's primary responsibility at an auto crash scene is to gain access to the vehicle and provide emergency medical care to the patient. The EMT cannot be both the person in charge of extrication and patient care. *(1.6.51)*

200.

D. When driving with lights and siren, you must always drive with due regard to others. The non-emergency vehicles must yield the right of way to an emergency vehicle. *(1.6.54)*

201.

C. If the patient begins complaining of other symptoms or if the symptom is worsening, you must re-assess by inspecting and palpating the involved area or relevant body system. *(1.6.57)*

7 Airway Management and Ventilation

chapter objectives

Questions in this chapter relate to DOT objectives 1.7.1–1.7.40. Please see the Appendix for more information.

DIRECTIONS Each of the questions or incomplete statements below is followed by suggested answers or completions. Select the **one answer** that is best in each case.

1. Damage or failure of which cardiovascular structure would cause an immediate decrease in perfusion of pulmonary capillaries?
   A. aorta
   B. coronary arteries
   C. pulmonary arteries
   D. pulmonary veins

2. A sign of a fractured larynx may be:
   A. aphagia.
   B. hypotension.
   C. subcutaneous emphysema.
   D. bradycardia.

3. A function of the epiglottis is to:
   A. prevent air from entering the esophagus.
   B. direct food into the thyroid opening.
   C. allow air to enter the esophagus during breathing.
   D. allow air to enter the trachea during inhalation.

4. Which of the following will cause a decrease in the PaO_2 level in the blood?
   A. lactic acidosis
   B. aerobic metabolism
   C. poorly saturated hemoglobin
   D. depressed metabolism

5. An increase in the production of CO_2 may be the result of:
   A. diminished respiratory rate.
   B. diminished metabolic rate.
   C. increased respiratory rate.
   D. increased metabolic rate.

6. You arrive on scene to find a 56-year-old male who is breathing deeply at 32 times a minute. During your assessment you find no subjective or objective indications of respiratory distress. What would you expect his $PaCO_2$ level to be?
   A. initially increased, then decreased
   B. initially decreased, then increased
   C. most likely lower than normal
   D. most likely higher than normal

7. All of the following statements about the purpose of suctioning are true, **except**:
   A. It can lower airway resistance during positive pressure ventilation.
   B. It can help remove excess fluid from the alveolar-capillary membrane.
   C. It can promote hypoxia if incorrectly performed.
   D. It can be safely performed on an infant.

8. What is the most effective way of unclogging a partially occluded suction catheter while performing oral suctioning?
   A. Disassemble the tip and clean manually.
   B. Increase the amount of suction applied.
   C. Aspirate water through the catheter.
   D. Strike the tip against a hard surface.

9. What is a disadvantage when using an esophageal obturator airway to manage the airway in a comatose patient?
   A. It does not isolate the stomach.
   B. It causes esophageal tissue necrosis upon insertion.
   C. It does not prevent the aspiration of fluids.
   D. It causes gastric distention when improperly used.

10. Which of the following mechanical airways or adjuncts should **not** be used for prolonged periods of time?
    A. nasopharyngeal airway
    B. oropharyngeal airway
    C. esophageal obturator airway
    D. endotracheal tube

11. What is the best way to detect the integrity of the esophageal balloon of a properly placed esophageal gastric tube airway?
    A. absence of gastric sounds during positive pressure ventilation
    B. good skin color
    C. inflated mask cuff
    D. inflated pilot balloon

12. What is the most common error found when using the esophageal obturator airway that makes it ineffective?
    A. inserting the device until the mask touches the face
    B. holding the mask seal poorly due to operator fatigue
    C. overinflating the esophageal balloon
    D. applying the face mask on upside down

13. Which of the following airways will always prevent aspiration if properly placed?
    A. endotracheal tube
    B. esophageal tracheal combitube
    C. pharyngeal tracheal lumen airway
    D. esophageal gastric tube airway

14. Skill deterioration can be best avoided by:
    A. intermittently assessing and treating a patient.
    B. reading EMS literature and practicing skills.
    C. reading the equipment manufacturer's instructions for the device.
    D. attend one EMS conference a year.

15. Which statement in regard to the anatomy of the upper airway is most accurate?
    A. The vallecula prevents food from entering the respiratory system while swallowing.
    B. The larynx joins the pharynx with the trachea.
    C. The larynx contains several openings such as the eustachian tube and the posterior nares.
    D. The thyroid cartilage, like the tracheal cartilages, forms a complete circle.

16. Which of the following statements about the vocal cords is true?
    A. The vocal cords are contained within the oropharynx.
    B. The vocal cords are found within the larynx.
    C. The vocal cords are housed within the cricoid cartilage.
    D. The vocal cords represent the opening into the esophagus.

17. Which of the following describes the relationship between the esophagus and the larynx:
    A. The larynx passes food while the esophagus passes water.
    B. The larynx and the esophagus exit at the same point.
    C. The larynx lies anterior to the esophagus.
    D. The larynx and the esophagus are comprised of cartilage.

18. CO_2 production increases with which of the following?
    A. fever
    B. hypoventilation
    C. carbon monoxide inhalation
    D. hyperventilation

19. Excess carbon dioxide (CO_2) is removed from the blood by:
    A. bradypnea and hypopnea.
    B. urinary excretion.
    C. tachypnea and hyperpnea.
    D. sweating.

20. Suctioning is a priority in emergency care to:
    A. prevent fluids from entering the esophagus.
    B. remove excess CO_2 from the respiratory system.
    C. prevent fluids from entering the trachea.
    D. reduce mucus production.

21. Which statement about suctioning is the most accurate?
    A. Suctioning should be limited to 30 seconds.
    B. Apply suction only during the insertion of the catheter.
    C. Oxygenation between suctioning attempts is not necessary.
    D. Suctioning should be limited to 10 seconds in the adult.

22. You have just place an esophageal obturator airway in a 77-year-old cardiac arrest patient. This method of airway control must be monitored carefully because?
    A. An esophageal obturator airway does not assure a patent airway.
    B. An esophageal obturator airway requires direct visualization of the esophagus.
    C. Gastric distention upon ventilation is a possibility.
    D. An esophageal obturator airway is effective only in cases of trauma.

23. Once the esophageal obturator airway is placed, how much air should be placed in the distal cuff?
    A. 10 cc
    B. 20 cc
    C. 25 cc
    D. 35 cc

24. You are treating an unconscious non-breathing 13-year-old male who was involved in a car crash. Endotracheal intubation equipment is not available. What is the best alternative for this patient?
    A. a nasal airway and supplemental oxygen
    B. a demand valve
    C. an oral airway and bag-valve-mask with an oxygen reservoir
    D. an esophageal obturator airway

25. You are treating a patient who needs to be intubated. All of the following statements about the endotracheal intubation process are true, **except**:
    A. It is important to place the endotracheal tube on the first attempt regardless of how long it takes.
    B. Each endotracheal attempt should be limited to 30 seconds.
    C. The patient should be hyperventilated before each attempt to place the endotracheal tube.
    D. During endotracheal intubation, hypoxia can result because of operator inexperience.

26. A physician informs you that the 54-year-old male you transported has a PaO_2 of 94 mmHg on room air. You know that this figure is considered:
    A. low.
    B. normal.

C. high.

D. extremely high.

27. Which of the following would be considered a normal PaCO$_2$?

A. 100 mmHg.

B. 49 mmHg.

C. 38 mmHg.

D. 75 mmHg.

28. Which of the following statements would most correctly describe a healthy individual's PaCO$_2$ level and respiratory status during exercise?

A. hypercarbic, increase in respiratory activity

B. hypocapnic, increase in respiratory activity

C. hypocarbic, increase in respiratory activity

D. hypercapnic, no change in respiratory activity

29. A healthy individual has inhaled a considerable amount of smoke and presents as cyanotic and restless. Which of the following statements would best describe the condition and the expected respiratory rate?

A. hypoxia, decrease in respirations

B. hypoxia, increase in respirations

C. hypercapnia, decrease in respirations

D. hypoxic drive, decrease in respirations

30. Which of the following statements best describes why airway control with an esophageal obturator airway is detrimental to any patient over 7 feet in height?

A. The inflatable cuff is too small for effective occlusion.

B. Direct visualization of the esophagus is required for proper placement.

C. There is greater opportunity for gastric distention and aspiration.

D. A greater possibility exists for tracheal occlusion.

31. A correctly placed esophageal obturator airway can be removed:

A. after endotracheal intubation.

B. when a pulse oximetry reading is greater than 95 percent.

C. after 1 hour of esophageal placement so as to avoid esophageal necrosis.

D. It is never permissible to remove an in-place esophageal obturator airway.

32. An esophageal tracheal combitube or a pharyngeal trachea lumen airway would be most beneficial in a(n):

A. semiconscious patient with severe shortness of breath.

B. unresponsive patient with severe posterior epistaxis.

C. unresponsive head injured patient with severe vomiting.

D. unresponsive patient who has ingested bleach.

33. Prior to esophageal obturator airway placement the EMT-Intermediate must have available:

A. suction, stylet, 35-cc syringe.

B. bag-valve-mask, stylet, oxygen source, oxygen tubing.

C. 35-cc syringe, laryngoscope, bag-valve-mask.

D. oxygen source, suction, lubricant, oral airway.

34. While ventilating a patient who has an endotracheal tube in place, you notice that the pilot balloon will not remain inflated. You would suspect:
    A. inadequate connection between the bag-valve-mask and the pilot balloon.
    B. the endotracheal tube has been mis-placed in the esophagus.
    C. increased airway resistance.
    D. a leaking tracheal cuff.

35. The best indicator of proper endotracheal tube placement would be:
    A. absence of epigastric ventilation sounds.
    B. adequate breath sounds.
    C. ease in bag-valve-mask compliance.
    D. visualization of the tube passing between the vocal cords.

36. Besides preventing inadvertent tube dis-lodgment, a properly placed endotracheal tube should be secured to prevent:
    A. the patient from biting down on the tube.
    B. laceration by the metal stylet.
    C. inadvertent cardiovascular stimulation.
    D. rupture of the pilot balloon.

37. The normal range for arterial $PaCO_2$ is:
    A. 15–25 mmHg.
    B. 25–35 mmHg.
    C. 35–45 mmHg.
    D. 45–55 mmHg.

38. What is the effect of hypercapnia on the res-piratory rate of a healthy individual?
    A. Respiratory rate and depth are unchanged.
    B. Respiratory rate increases while the depth is unchanged.
    C. Respiratory rate decreases while the depth is unchanged.
    D. Respiratory rate and depth increase.

39. What is the effect of hypocapnia on the res-piratory rate of a healthy individual?
    A. Respiratory rate and depth are unchanged.
    B. Respiratory rate increases while the depth is unchanged.
    C. Respiratory rate decreases while the depth is unchanged.
    D. Respiratory rate and depth increases.

40. Possible causes of increased CO_2 production include:
    A. asthma and respiratory depression.
    B. fever and shivering.
    C. head injury and drug overdose.
    D. airway obstruction and paralysis of the respiratory muscles.

41. It would be appropriate to remove an esophageal obturator airway if:
    A. an endotracheal tube is inserted.
    B. it has been in place for 1 hour.
    C. suctioning is required.
    D. excessive secretions are noted.

42. All of the following are advantages of an esophageal obturator airway **except**:
    A. the esophageal obturator airway prevents gastric distention and regurgitation.
    B. visualization is not required for insertion.
    C. esophageal intubation can be accom-plished by untrained personnel.
    D. insertion can be accomplished without hyperextension.

43. An oropharyngeal airway is an effective air-way adjunct because it prevents the tongue from obstructing the airway and it:
    A. isolates the trachea.
    B. allows air to pass around and through the device.

C. is flexible and fits the airway.

D. will not stimulate vomiting.

44. Prior to inserting an esophageal obturator airway, you should first hyperventilate the patient and then:

A. place the patient in the sniffing position.

B. hyperextend the patient's head and neck.

C. flex the patient's head slightly forward.

D. elevate the patient's shoulders with padding.

45. Which of the following is a relative contraindication of endotracheal intubation?

A. ingestion of a caustic substance

B. major facial and neck trauma

C. esophageal varices

D. spinal injury

46. Complications associated with suctioning include hypoxia, vagal stimulation, and:

A. improved airway patency.

B. hyperventilation.

C. soft tissue injury.

D. hyperoxygenation.

47. Which anatomical structure is responsible for regulating the passage of air through the larynx?

A. vocal cords

B. epiglottis

C. arytenoid folds

D. lesser cornu

48. Which anatomic structure lies directly posterior to the cricoid cartilage?

A. hyoid bone

B. esophagus

C. vallecula

D. epiglottis

49. Which of the following statements regarding the esophageal opening and its structure is true?

A. The esophageal opening is surrounded by cartilaginous structures.

B. The esophageal structure is positioned posterior to the larynx.

C. The esophageal structure is supported by semi-circular cartilage.

D. The esophageal opening is protected from food by the epiglottis.

50. Which cartilaginous body prevents food from entering the respiratory tract during the act of swallowing?

A. thyroid cartilage

B. epiglottis cartilage

C. cricoid cartilage

D. tracheal cartilage

51. To visualize the glottic opening when performing direct laryngoscopy, you must first lift which structure?

A. vocal cords

B. hyoid bone

C. vocal fold

D. epiglottis

52. The most common cause of airway obstruction is:

A. the tongue blocking the airway

B. a foreign body obstruction

C. aspiration of vomitus or food

D. laryngeal spasm constriction

53. Loss of muscle tone to which muscle may cause the tongue to fall back against the pharynx causing an occluded airway?

A. rectus femoris muscle

B. vastus lateralis muscle

C. submandibular muscle

D. gastrocnemius muscle

54. Which of the following structures is the primary landmark for insertion of an endotracheal tube?

    A. tracheal cartilage
    B. aryepiglottic fold
    C. false vocal cords
    D. true vocal cords

55. All of the following statements about the technique of suctioning are true, **except**:

    A. the tonsil tip catheter is used to suction the lower airway.
    B. each suctioning attempt should be limited to 10 seconds.
    C. suction is applied only when withdrawing the catheter.
    D. serious cardiac dysrhythmias can occur during suctioning.

56. To help prevent viscous secretions from obstructing the suction tubing, you should:

    A. reverse the suction action to help expel the thick secretions.
    B. suction water through the tubing between suctioning attempts.
    C. pre-treat the tubing before suctioning with a petroleum lubricant.
    D. replace the suction tubing between every suctioning attempt.

57. You are about to suction a patient's mouth and oropharynx using the soft (French) catheter. Which is the proper way to measure the catheter?

    A. Measure from the patient's corner of the mouth to the tip of their ear.
    B. Measure form the tip of the patient's nose to the tip of their ear.
    C. Measure the length of the patient's little finger then multiply by two.
    D. Measure from the corner of the patient's mouth to the thyroid cartilage.

58. A limitation of the battery-powered suction unit is:

    A. the unit becomes ineffective when the battery runs out.
    B. the unit requires two trained personnel to operate effectively.
    C. the suction created is too strong to use on infants and children.
    D. this suction device is limited to the confines of the ambulance.

59. Which type of suction unit is more effective when suctioning heavier, tenacious substances?

    A. engine manifold powered unit
    B. oxygen powered unit
    C. electric powered unit
    D. hand powered unit

60. All of the following statements about the use of the rigid suction catheter are correct, **except**:

    A. The rigid suction catheter is used to suction the mouth of unresponsive patients.
    B. The rigid suction catheter is inserted into the mouth only as far as you can see.
    C. The rigid suction catheter is not used to suction the back of the airway of infants.
    D. The rigid suction catheter is used to suction the laryngopharynx and glottic space.

61. The purpose of the distal cuff on the esophageal obturator airway is to:

    A. prevent regurgitation by blocking the trachea.
    B. provide a seal between the mask and the face.
    C. secure the tube in place by using direct contact.
    D. block the esophagus and prevents vomiting.

62. When preparing to insert the esophageal obturator airway you must have which of the following equipment ready?
    A. 10-cc syringe, suction unit, laryngoscope and blades, metal stylet
    B. 20-cc syringe, suction unit, laryngoscope and blades, stethoscope
    C. 25-cc syringe, suction unit, water-soluble lubricant, lighted stylet
    D. 35-cc syringe, suction unit, water-soluble lubricant, stethoscope

63. Which of the following is not a desired feature of the bag-valve-mask?
    A. pop-off valve
    B. self-refilling bag
    C. transparent mask
    D. oxygen reservoir

64. Which of the following patients should **not** be intubated by orotracheal intubation?
    A. an unresponsive overdose patient who will not tolerate an oropharyngeal airway
    B. an unresponsive cardiac patient who does not respond to any type of stimulus
    C. a respiratory patient who becomes unresponsive to voice and tactile stimulation
    D. an unresponsive trauma patient who has copious amounts of blood in the airway

65. If after placing the endotracheal tube you are unsure if the tube is properly placed, you should:
    A. remove the tube and immediately attempt to reintubate the patient.
    B. deflate the cuff and gently withdraw the tube 1 to 2 cm and recheck.
    C. immediately remove the tube and ventilate using a oropharyngeal airway and a bag-valve-mask.

D. when unsure if the tube is properly placed, have your partner reassess.

66. All of the following are potential complications of endotracheal suctioning, **except**:
    A. hypoxia may result from a decrease in lung air volume.
    B. cardiac arrhythmias may occur from suctioning the airway.
    C. bronchospasm may occur from insertion past the carina.
    D. stimulating the back of the throat may cause bradycardia.

67. All of the following are located in the pharynx, **except**:
    A. epiglottis
    B. gag reflex nerves
    C. vallecula
    D. vocal cords

68. You are called to manage a patient who has ingested a narcotic. Ingestion of narcotics can result in:
    A. hypocapnia.
    B. hypernatremia.
    C. respiratory acidosis.
    D. respiratory alkalosis.

69. Increased levels of $PaCO_2$ result in:
    A. polyuria.
    B. hyperventilation.
    C. hypoventilation.
    D. hypoxia.

70. Which of the following increases the production of carbon dioxide?
    A. airway obstruction
    B. asthma
    C. fever
    D. narcotic drugs

71. Respiratory alkalosis results when:
    A. carbon dioxide is eliminated, resulting in the loss of hydrogen ions and an increase in pH.
    B. carbon dioxide is eliminated, resulting in an increase of hydrogen ions and an increase in pH.
    C. carbon dioxide is retained, resulting in the loss of hydrogen ions and an increase in pH.
    D. carbon dioxide is retained, resulting in an increase of hydrogen ions and an increase in pH.

72. Which of the following is an advantage of the esophageal obturator airway?
    A. The esophageal obturator airway completely isolates the trachea.
    B. The esophageal obturator airway can be inserted on a conscious patient.
    C. The esophageal obturator airway prevents regurgitation and gastric distention.
    D. The esophageal obturator airway provides a direct route to the respiratory passages.

73. Which of the following airway adjuncts completely isolates the trachea, assuring a patent airway?
    A. oropharyngeal airway
    B. nasopharyngeal airway
    C. endotracheal tube
    D. esophageal obturator airway

74. You have inserted an esophageal obturator airway into your patient. You note that there is no chest rise, and on auscultation of lung fields, you do not detect any sounds. However, you do hear gurgling sounds over the epigastrium. You should:

A. attach the mask and begin ventilation.
B. inflate the cuff with 35 cc of air or until you have met resistance.
C. withdraw the airway approximately 2 cm as you have inserted it too deeply.
D. withdraw the airway and attempt insertion again as you have placed it in the trachea.

75. The appropriate equipment for intubating an infant is:
    A. a curved laryngoscope blade and cuffed endotracheal tube.
    B. a curved laryngoscope blade and uncuffed endotracheal tube.
    C. a straight laryngoscope blade and cuffed endotracheal tube.
    D. a straight laryngoscope blade and uncuffed endotracheal tube.

76. All of the following are alternative airway adjuncts to endotracheal intubation for the apneic patient, **except**:
    A. nasogastric tube airway.
    B. esophageal gastric tube airway.
    C. pharyngeal tracheal lumen airway.
    D. esophageal tracheal combitube airway.

77. Select the statement that best describes the relationship between the epiglottis and the larynx.
    A. The larynx is superior to the epiglottis.
    B. The epiglottis is superior to the larynx.
    C. The epiglottis is at the same level as the larynx.
    D. The epiglottis is inferior to the larynx.

78. Select the statement that best describes the relationship between the tongue and the larynx?

A. The tongue is superior and anterior to the larynx.

B. The tongue is inferior and anterior to the larynx.

C. The tongue is inferior and posterior to the larynx.

D. The tongue is superior and posterior to the larynx.

79. The anterior portion of the larynx that forms a "V" shape is called the:

A. thyroid cartilage.

B. anterior cartilage.

C. Adam's apple.

D. cricoid cartilage.

80. What is the relationship between the false vocal cords and the true vocal cords?

A. The false cords are inferior to the true cords.

B. The false cords are lateral to the true cords.

C. The false cords are medial to the true cords.

D. The false cords are located in the oropharynx.

81. What is the space between the vocal cords called?

A. septum

B. vallecula

C. pyriform fossa

D. glottis

82. Which statement best describes the relationship of the pharynx to the larynx?

A. The larynx is anterior to the pharynx.

B. The larynx is posterior to the pharynx.

C. The larynx is inferior to the pharynx.

D. The larynx is superior to the pharynx.

83. What is the most superior region of the pharynx called?

A. hyperpharynx

B. oropharynx

C. nasopharynx

D. laryngopharynx

84. Which of the following is a normal arterial blood oxygen concentration (PaO_2)?

A. 50 mmHg

B. 60 mmHg

C. 70 mmHg

D. 90 mmHg

85. Which of the following is **not** a common method used to develop negative pressure in an adult suction unit?

A. engine manifold power

B. electrical powered

C. hand- or foot-powered

D. mouth-powered

86. Two of the most common types of suction catheters used in prehospital care are:

A. whistle tip and standard tip.

B. whistle tip and tonsil tip.

C. tonsil tip and standard tip.

D. tonsil tip and Yankauer tip.

87. Which statement best describes a whistle tip (soft) suction catheter?

A. a rigid tube with two openings on the distal end

B. a part rigid and part flexible tube with two openings on the distal end

C. a long flexible tube with an open distal end

D. a rigid tube with three openings on the distal end

88. You are ventilating a patient in respiratory arrest with a bag-valve-mask device. The patient suddenly vomits. What type of suction catheter should you select?

    A. whistle-tip suction catheter
    B. standard-tip suction catheter
    C. tonsil-tip suction catheter
    D. miller-tip suction catheter

89. What type of catheter would you use for tracheal suctioning?

    A. soft suction catheter
    B. standard-tip suction catheter
    C. tonsil-tip suction catheter
    D. miller-tip suction catheter

90. Which of the following is an indication for the use of the esophageal tracheal combitube airway?

    A. a patient with an intact gag reflex who requires ventilation
    B. a patient with respirations of 4 per minute and significant bleeding in the oropharynx
    C. a patient in respiratory arrest who ingested a caustic substance.
    D. an adult trauma patient in whom you are unable to place an endotracheal tube

91. All of the following items should be available prior to placing an ETC airway, **except**:

    A. stethoscope.
    B. water-soluble lubricant.
    C. 35-cc syringe.
    D. stylet.

92. Select the sequence for insertion of the esophageal obturator airway. Your partner is hyperventilating the patient while you prepare to place the device.

    1. Ventilate and verify tube placement.
    2. Place the patient's head in the neutral position.
    3. With mask attached, insert the tube.
    4. Inflate the cuff.
    5. Check the equipment and distal cuff.

    A. 5, 2, 3, 1, 4
    B. 2, 5, 3, 1, 4
    C. 5, 2, 3, 4, 1
    D. 2, 5, 1, 3, 4

93. All of the following statements about the placement of the esophageal obturator airway are false, **except**:

    A. place the head in a flexed position prior to insertion.
    B. place the head in an extended position prior to insertion.
    C. inflate the cuff and then verify tube placement.
    D. verify tube placement and then inflate the cuff.

94. What is the most common cause of poor ventilation in a patient with an esophageal obturator airway?

    A. failure to connect oxygen to the bag-valve-mask
    B. failure to inflate the distal balloon on the esophageal obturator airway
    C. failure to provide an adequate ventilation rate
    D. failure to maintain a tight mask to face seal

95. In which patient could the esophageal obturator airway be utilized?

    A. a patient who is 16 years of age
    B. a patient under 5 feet or over 6 feet, 7 inches tall
    C. a patient who ingested a caustic poison
    D. a patient with a history of esophageal disease or alcoholism

96. An unresponsive trauma patient in respiratory arrest is trapped in a sitting position in

a wrecked vehicle. There is limited maneuvering room in the vehicle. It is the middle of the day and the patient is located in direct sunlight. Which technique of endotracheal intubation is most appropriate for this situation?

A. orotracheal intubation

B. nasotracheal intubation

C. transillumination intubation

D. digital intubation

97. Which of the following actions would best prevent deterioration of airway management skills?

A. Constantly read and review your textbook.

B. Watch a videotape reviewing the procedure.

C. Practice the skills on a continual basis.

D. Listen to an audio tape describing the procedures.

98. Endotracheal intubation must be accomplished within:

A. 30 seconds.

B. 40 seconds.

C. 50 seconds.

D. 60 seconds.

99. A 13-year-old female patient witnessed her pet getting hit and killed by a car. She now presents to you with classic indications of stress-induced hyperventilation syndrome. You would expect her carbon dioxide levels to be:

A. diminished because of increased alveolar ventilation.

B. increased because of the extra acid production from breathing so hard.

C. diminished because of the levels of oxygen in her blood stream rising from the increased ventilation.

D. increased because of the drop in alveolar ventilation.

100. All of the following statements regarding suctioning are correct, **except**:

A. routine suctioning should not take longer than 5 to 10 seconds per episode.

B. you should not suction infants because of the inherent danger of hypoxemia.

C. prolonged suctioning may precipitate hypoxemia.

D. application of suction to the suction tip should only occur while the catheter is being removed.

101. All of the following statements regarding the portable suction machine are true, **except**:

A. the collection bottle should be cleaned and disinfected after use.

B. improper assembly of the equipment may cause the unit to fail next time it is needed.

C. the unit should be left charging in between calls.

D. the device is not designed to be used with a French-tip catheter.

102. The EMT-I should exercise caution whenever using the esophageal obturator airway (EOA) because:

A. the pharyngeal cuff may leak, rendering the device useless.

B. it may cause oral mucosal damage during insertion.

C. it does not prevent possible aspiration.

D. all of the above

103. At what level of the airway does occlusion occur when the tongue relaxes and falls against the back of the throat in an unresponsive patient?
    A. nasopharynx
    B. oropharynx
    C. hypopharynx
    D. laryngopharynx

104. Which of the following pieces of equipment is not always necessary during endotracheal intubation of an adult patient with apnea and no gag reflex?
    A. a 10-ml syringe
    B. a #3 or #4 Miller straight blade
    C. a malleable stylet
    D. a laryngoscope handle

105. Of the following types of continuing education involving endotracheal intubation, which one is most helpful for the EMT-I?
    A. watching a video on intubation
    B. listening to a lecture on intubation
    C. reading a review manual on intubation
    D. practicing the skill of intubation on a mannequin

106. During the process of intubation, when should the endotracheal tube stop being advanced?
    A. when the proximal end of the cuff passes through the true vocal cords
    B. when the proximal end of the cuff passes along side the false vocal cords
    C. when the distal end of the cuff passes through the true vocal cords
    D. when the distal end of the cuff passes alongside the false vocal cords

107. What airway structure houses the vocal cords?
    A. pharynx
    B. larynx
    C. epiglottis
    D. carina

108. Of the following list of PaO_2 values, which one represents a normal value for a patient with no respiratory compromise?
    A. 35 mmHg
    B. 58 mmHg
    C. 72 mmHg
    D. 88 mmHg

109. Of the following list of $PaCO_2$ values, which one represents a normal value for a patient with no respiratory compromise?
    A. 35 mmHg
    B. 58 mmHg
    C. 72 mmHg
    D. 88 mmHg

110. Which of the following situations is a contraindication to the insertion of an EOA for an unresponsive patient?
    A. absence of a gag reflex
    B. ingestion of a caustic substance
    C. a patient who is 5¢11≤ tall, weighing 122 pounds
    D. history of gastric ulcers

111. Which one of the following airways, when properly inserted, could still allow for aspiration of foreign material into the trachea?
    A. esophageal tracheal combitube
    B. pharyngeotracheal lumen airway
    C. esophageal obturator airway
    D. all of the above

112. As you are transporting a patient with severe pulmonary edema, your partner states that the patient's trachea needs suctioning. The most correct statement is:

A. tracheal suctioning should not be completed in the prehospital phase.

B. the trachea could be suctioned, but only by an EMT-Paramedic.

C. the trachea could be suctioned, but not for longer than 20 seconds at a time.

D. the trachea could be suctioned, but use lower levels of suction than pharyngeal suctioning.

113. What advantage does placement of an esophageal obturator airway (EOA) have over an oropharyngeal airway (OPA) in the airway maintenance of an unresponsive patient?

A. It will prevent aspiration of blood.

B. It will prevent regurgitation.

C. It can be used in a patient with an intact gag reflex.

D. none of the above

114. Which of the following statements about the esophageal obturator airway is true?

A. It provides a route for drug therapy into the lungs.

B. The insertion of the device is a blind technique.

C. You do not need to implement a manual airway technique after insertion.

D. It does not rely on a mask to work properly.

115. What would be the best indication that the esophageal obturator airway should be removed?

A. return of spontaneous ventilations

B. cessation of gastric regurgitation

C. return of the gag-reflex

D. arrival at the emergency department

116. While checking out the ambulance supplies at the beginning of the shift, your EMT-Basic partner asks you what the little holes near the proximal end of the esophageal tube of the EOA are for. How would you reply?

A. They allow air to escape from the stomach.

B. They allow the patient to be ventilated via the trachea.

C. They allow access to the hypopharynx for suctioning.

D. none of the above

117. Vocal cords are responsible for speech and are located:

A. in the larynx.

B. in the trachea.

C. in the carina.

D. in the hyoid bone.

118. Which one of the following clinical indications would alert you to a possible misplaced endotracheal tube?

A. noticeable abdominal distention

B. a decrease in bagging resistance

C. moisture inside the lumen of the endotracheal tube

D. high carbon dioxide reading in the end-tidal CO_2 monitor

119. The trachea bifurcates into the right and left mainstem bronchus at the:

A. glottis.

B. aretynoid.

C. carina.

D. hypopharynx.

120. When placing an endotracheal tube or esophageal tracheal combitube in the trachea, the tube must first pass:
    A. between the esophagus and larynx.
    B. through the glottic opening and between the vocal cords.
    C. behind the vocal cords and through the larynx.
    D. through the crocoid cartilage and between the thyroid cartilage.

121. The esophagus is located:
    A. inferior to the larynx.
    B. anterior to the thryroid cartilage.
    C. superior to the aretynoid catfilage.
    D. posterior to the glottic opening.

122. A patient begins to choke and gasp for air while drinking a glass of water. Which of the following structures are most likely involved in this event?
    A. epiglottis and vocal cords
    B. esophagus and cricoid cartilage
    C. thyroid cartilage and epiglottis
    D. trachea and bronchus

123. Which of the following structures is common to both the esophagus and laryngeal opening?
    A. carina
    B. pharynx
    C. stomach
    D. diaphragm

124. You arrive on the scene and find a 26-year-old male patient who is visibly upset because of the breakup with his girlfriend. He is complaining of tingling in his extremities, lightheadedness, and a tightness in his chest. His BP is 138/66, HR is 96/minute, and respirations are 46/minute and deep and full. If an arterial blood gas sample was drawn, what would you expect the PaO_2 level to be?
    A. greater than 100 mmHg
    B. 80–90 mmHg
    C. 35–45 mmHg
    D. less than 40 mmHg

125. You have been hyperventilating a respiratory failure patient with a bag-valve-mask device connected to supplemental oxygen at 15 lpm for the last 30 minutes during transport to the emergency department. What would you expect the arterial blood gases to be upon arrival?
    A. PaO_2 less than 40 mmHg, $PaCO_2$ greater than 100 mmHg
    B. PaO_2 of 100 mmHg, $PaCO_2$ of 40 mmHg
    C. PaO_2 greater than 100 mmHg, $PaCO_2$ less than 35 mmHg
    D. PaO_2 less than 100 mmHg, $PaCO_2$ greater than 40 mmHg

126. As the $PaCO_2$ level rises in the normal person, the:
    A. pH will be greater than 7.40 and the respirations will increase.
    B. pH will be less than 7.40 and the respirations will increase.
    C. pH will not be affected and respirations will decrease.
    D. pH will be greater than 7.40 and the respirations will increase.

127. In response to hypoxia, the chemoreceptors will stimulate the respiratory center to:
    A. increase the respiratory rate and depth.
    B. decrease the respiratory rate and depth.
    C. decrease the heart rate.
    D. increase the respiratory depth only.

128. You arrive on the scene and find a patient who has a large contusion to his head from

a fall down a flight of steps. He displays decorticate posturing to painful stimuli. His BP is 192/68 mmHg, HR is 56/minute, and RR is 42/minute and shallow. What would you expect the patient's arterial blood gases to be?

A. $PaO_2 > 100$ mmHg, $PaCO_2 < 40$ mmHg

B. PaO_2 80 mmHg, $PaCO_2$ 35 mmHg

C. $PaO_2 < 90$ mmHg, $PaCO_2 > 45$ mmHg

D. $PaO_2 < 80$ mmHg, $PaCO_2 < 40$ mmHg

129. Based on the patient's condition you determine that you need to decrease the $PaCO_2$ level. What would be the most effective method to do this?

A. Infuse about 250 to 500 ml of normal saline.

B. Administer lasix to increase the urine output.

C. Apply a nonrebreather mask at 15 lpm.

D. Ventilate the patient at a rate of 24/minute.

130. You arrive on scene and find a patient who appears to be unresponsive on the floor in the kitchen. The family states the patient began slurring his words and complained of a severe headache followed by unconsciousness. You find the patient supine, with vomitus coming from his mouth and apparently not breathing. Which of the following would be your next immediate action?

A. Check for a pulse.

B. Suction the airway and perform a head-tilt chin-lift maneuver.

C. Begin bag-valve-mask ventilation with supplemental oxygen.

D. Suction the airway and apply a nonrebreather mask at 15 lpm.

131. You are treating a patient with an altered mental status who is not breathing. You have suctioned the oropharynx and have inserted an oropharyngeal airway. The patient has a large amount of vomitus in both nostrils. Which of the following would be your next action?

A. Begin bag-valve-mask ventilation with supplemental oxygen.

B. Immediately insert a ETC combitube or PTL airway.

C. Insert a nasopharyngeal airway in the right nasopharynx.

D. Suction both nasopharyngeal passages with a soft suction catheter.

132. Which of the following would best describe the purpose for insertion of an esophageal obturator airway (EOA)?

A. The EOA will prevent regurgitation of gastric contents.

B. The EOA is the most effective means to ventilate a patient.

C. Regular bag-valve-mask ventilation is usually not effective when ventilating patients.

D. There is less fatigue associated with the EOA since a mask seal is not necessary.

133. You are treating a patient with a suspected ruptured esophageal varicies. There is a massive amount of blood in the airway. The patient is completely unresponsive and not breathing. You should immediately:

A. suction the airway, insert an EOA, and begin ventialtion.

B. turn the patient on his side, apply suction, and begin bag-valve-mask ventilation.

C. insert a nasopharyngeal airway and begin ventilation with a flow-restricted oxygen powered ventilation device.

D. place the patient in a prone position, apply a non-rebreather mask at 15 lpm, and transport immediately.

134. Which of the following is a major disadvantage of using the EOA?
    A. It cannot be used in patients greater than 5 feet tall.
    B. It does not prevent regurgitation in the unresponsive patient.
    C. It requires that a good mask seal and a manual airway maneuver be maintained.
    D. High concentrations of oxygen cannot be effectively delivered.

135. Which of the following is the most common problem associated with the EOA?
    A. insertion of the tube into the stomach
    B. inadequate ventilation caused by poor mask seal
    C. rupture of the trachea caused by improper insertion
    D. laryngospasm from tracheal intubation

136. Which of the following is **not** an advantage of an endotracheal tube?
    A. Drugs can be administered down the endotracheal tube.
    B. The endotracheal tube prevents aspiration of oral and nasal secretions.
    C. Oral intubation requires a laryngoscope and knowledge of the upper airway anatomy.
    D. It can be inserted around esophageal devices.

137. You arrive on scene and find a 56-year-old male patient who was involved in a motor vehicle crash. He has a significant amount of facial trauma from striking the windshield. You suction the airway but the mouth readily fills with blood again. How would you control the airway in this patient?
    A. Continue to suction and insert an oropharyngeal airway.
    B. Insert an esophageal obturator airway.
    C. Put the patient in a lateral recumbent position and perform a jaw-thrust maneuver.
    D. Insert an endotracheal tube.

138. Which of the following statements about endotracheal intubation is true?
    A. Skill maintenance requires continuous practice of laryngoscopy and review of upper airway anatomy.
    B. The preferred technique of insertion of the endotracheal tube is a blind technique that requires little skill.
    C. Because of the highly skillled procedure, only physicians should be allowed to intubate patients.
    D. Endotracheal intubation should only be performed on patients in cardiac arrest.

139. Which of the following is the best method to ensure you have properly placed the endotracheal tube?
    A. Auscultate the lungs for breath sounds and the stomach for gastric sounds.
    B. Look for a decrease in the oxygen saturation level on the pulse oximeter.
    C. Perform a laryngoscopy and directly visualize the tube in the glottic opening.
    D. Apply an esophageal tube check device.

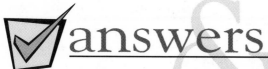
answers & rationales

1.

C. The pulmonary arteries transport blood from the right ventricle to the lungs for oxygenation. If a failure occurs here (such as a pulmonary emboli), blood will not reach the lungs for oxygenation. *(1.7.3)*

2.

C. A fractured larynx can allow air to escape into the soft tissues of the neck and upper chest, causing subcutaneous emphysema. Since it is a relatively avascular area, hypotension is not a concern nor is bradycardia. Aphagia is the inability to swallow. *(1.7.1A)*

3.

D. The epiglottis is a flap-like structure which uncovers the glottic opening during inhalation, thereby allowing inhaled air to gain access to the lungs. It closes over the top of the glottic opening during swallowing so that the material is directed into the esophagus. *(1.7.2C)*

4.

C. Arterial oxygen saturations decrease when there is a problem with oxygenation of the blood. This results in poorly saturated hemoglobin. Aerobic metabolism is cellular activity in the presence of oxygen and lactic acidosis is a byproduct of anaerobic metabolism. *(1.7.6)*

5.

D. Heightened metabolic activity is a common cause of elevated CO_2 levels as the cells of the body produce more waste products. A diminished respiratory rate may result in heightened CO_2 levels, but it is a function of diminished elimination and not increased production. Diminishment of the metabolic rate or elevations in the respiratory activity will both lower CO_2 levels. *(1.7.7)*

6.

C. His $PaCO_2$ would be lower than normal because the arterial level of carbon dioxide are a direct function of alveolar ventilation in the healthy person. An increase in alveolar ventilation will reduce the $PaCO_2$ levels in the bloodstream as it is eliminated at a faster rate through the lungs. *(1.7.8)*

7.

B. It is impossible to suction fluid from the capillary/alveolar membrane. At this level, the structures are much smaller than even a millimeter! Suctioning a patient either removes material from the pharynx or lower in the trachea if the patient has an endotracheal tube placed. *(1.7.9)*

8.

C. When a suction catheter becomes clogged, try suctioning water through the tip. This will often remove the clog. If that does not work, replace the tip. *(1.7.13)*

9.

C. An EOA does not prevent other material from entering the trachea, so the patient may still aspirate fluid that originates from the pharynx or oral cavity. Proper placement of an EOA only isolates the esophagus, decreasing the likelihood of regurgitation. It may also cause esophageal wall necrosis, but that is after more than 2 hours of placement. *(1.7.17)*

10.

C. Placement of the EOA in the esophagus can cause necrosis of the esophageal wall from the cuff. This condition is called "pressure necrosis." It is caused by the inflated cuff forcing the blood from the small capillary beds of the esophageal wall. An EOA should not be in place for longer than 2 hours at a time. *(1.7.18)*

11.

D. After the EGTA is placed, it is impossible to visually see if the esophageal cuff is inflated. To correct this, there is a pilot balloon positioned just distal to the inflation port—it stays inflated as long as cuff integrity is not lost. The mask balloon is separate from the esophageal balloon and is inflated by a different port. The other two answers suggest proper placement, but do not guarantee an inflated cuff. *(1.7.16)*

12.

B. The EOA only occludes the esophagus, it does not guarantee that the airway is open. To assure this, the EMT-I *must* reimplement a manual airway technique in order to remove the tongue from the posterior pharyngeal wall and hold a tight mask seal continuously. Because of its design, the mask cannot be put on upside down and overinflating the cuff only dilates the esophagus more. The mask is supposed to touch the face, so it also cannot be the reason for failure. *(1.7.26)*

13.

A. An endotracheal tube is the only airway that, after its proper placement, will always isolate the trachea from any material in the pharynx. The other three airways (ETC, Ptl, and EGTA) could be successfully placed in the esophagus but the trachea is still subject to aspiration. *(1.7.18)*

14.

B. Skill deterioration is a common problem for care providers in a low-volume EMS system. To avoid this, the EMT-I must take time to keep up with read-ing, and it is imperative to constantly practice your skills. Treating patients often will also decrease skill deterioration. *(1.7.31)*

15.

B. The larynx is the structure that joins the pharynx with the trachea. The pharynx or throat extends from the back of the soft palate to the esophagus and larynx. The pharynx contains the openings for the eustachian tube and posterior nares. The epiglottis is the structure that prevents food from entering the respiratory tract. The vallecula is just above the epiglottis. The thyroid and tracheal cartilages are open on their posterior surfaces, whereas the cricoid cartilage forms a complete ring. *(1.7.1)*

16.

B. The vocal cords are found within the larynx. They are actually housed within the thyroid cartilages, which is a part of the larynx. Anatomically, the vocal cords represent the opening into the trachea, not the esophagus. *(1.7.2a)*

17.

C. In terms of location, the larynx is anterior to the esophagus. The larynx and esophagus are separate structures that each serve a different function. The larynx is constructed of cartilage and is a conductor of air while the esophagus is soft and transports food and water into the stomach. *(1.7.2b)*

18.

A. A fever increases the metabolic rate of the cells in an attempt to speed up defensive actions and repair processes. Since water and carbon dioxide are waste products of aerobic cellular metabolism, an increase in cellular metabolism equates to an increase in waste products. Hypoventilation and hyperventilation are mechanisms that deal with the excretion or retention of CO_2, not the actual production. Carbon monoxide would pertain to displaced oxygen molecules and a switch to anaerobic cellular metabolism. Anaerobic metabolism yields lactic acid as a waste product, not CO_2 and H_2O. *(1.7.7)*

19.

C. Tachypnea, fast respirations, and deep breathing, hyperpnea, enhance alveolar ventilation and quickly "blow off" excessive amounts of carbon dioxide. Slow respirations would be ineffective in ventilating the excess CO_2 from the alveoli. Carbon dioxide is not excreted in the urine and sweat. *(1.7.8)*

20.

C. Securing a patent airway is always the priority in emergency care. Suctioning fluids from the airway is one of many ways to accomplish this task. The fluids are removed, thus preventing them from entering the trachea and ultimately the lungs. Suctioning has little effect on removing CO_2 and does not decrease mucus production. *(1.7.9)*

21.

D. Suctioning should be limited to 10 seconds in an adult. When possible the patient should be hyperventilated with 100 percent oxygen before and between each suctioning attempt. Suction should only be applied once the catheter is properly positioned and during withdrawal. *(1.7.10)*

22.

A. The esophageal obturator airway does not assure a patent airway because it is placed into the esophagus. An esophageal obturator airway does not protect the trachea from upper airway obstructions or secretions. Placement of the esophageal obturator airway is generally blind and does not require visualization of the esophagus. If the esophageal obturator airway is properly placed, it prevents gastric distention and regurgitation. The esophageal obturator airway is not limited to cases of trauma but can be used in medical emergencies as well. *(1.7.23)*

23.

D. The distal cuff should be inflated with 30 to 35 cc of air once the esophageal obturator airway is placed and the patient's chest rises and falls. Check the pilot balloon to verify inflation of the cuff. *(1.7.24)*

24.

C. The oral airway and the bag-valve-mask are the best alternative for the patient in this scenario. The esophageal obturator airway and the demand valve resuscitator are not recommended in patients under the age of 16. A nasal airway would be acceptable if the patient did not accept an oral airway, however in a non-breathing unconscious patient an oral airway should be attempted. The bag-valve-mask is necessary for high flow oxygen therapy and for assisting ventilations. The oral airway and bag-valve-mask both come in pediatric sizes. *(1.7.30)*

25.

A. Endotracheal intubation requires trained personnel and intubation efforts should not be a lengthy process. Hypoxia can occur from oxygen delays and operator inexperience. The patient should be hyperventilated before and after each attempt, and each attempt should be limited to 30 seconds. *(1.7.32)*

26.

B. While the optimal figure for arterial oxygen is 100 mmHg, the range 80 to 100 mmHg is considered within normal limits. This patient has a PO_2 measured at 94 mmHg, which falls within the suggested range and is not an immediate concern. *(1.7.3)*

27.

C. The average range of normal $PaCO_2$ values spans 35 to 45 mmHg. 38 mmHg is within this range and is therefore considered normal. *(1.7.4)*

28.

A. During exertion, activity at the cellular level increases in an effort to meet the added demand. This heightened cellular activity results in an increase in the byproducts of water and CO_2. The $PaCO_2$ would increase and be described as hypercarbic. In an effort to rid itself of the added waste products, the neuroregulatory system increases respiratory activity so as to excrete the CO_2 via pulmonary ventilation. *(1.7.5)*

29.

B. This individual has experienced a drop in arterial oxygen saturation caused by the toxic inhalation and is therefore hypoxic. In an effort to get more oxygen the respiratory centers in the brain will increase the respiratory activity. Hypercapnia refers to the retention of CO_2 and the hypoxic drive refers to individuals who have lost their ability to regulate internal CO_2 levels and breath in accordance to their PaO_2—such is as seen with COPD patients. *(1.7.6)*

30.

D. To be effective, an esophageal obturator airway must occlude the esophagus at a level lower than the carina. An individual of 7 feet in height or greater would most likely have a longer trachea and placement of the one sized esophageal obturator airway would locate the cuff directly behind the trachea. Because the posterior wall of the trachea is quite flexible, inflation of the cuff with 35 cc of air could push the esophogeal cuff into the tracheal lumen creating an airway occlusion. *(1.7.15)*

31.

A. An esophageal obturator airway can be appropriately removed after an endotracheal tube has been correctly placed. An esophageal obturator airway should never be removed based solely on the pulse oximetry reading. *(1.7.16)*

32.

C. The unresponsive head injured patient who is vomiting would benefit most from the placement of an airway adjunct. A semiconscious patient would most likely have an intact gag reflex that could precipitate vomiting if stimulated. These devices should never be utilized when caustic ingestion has occurred. *(1.7.17)*

33.

D. An oxygen source, suction, lubricant, and an oral airway are included among the items that an EMT-Intermediate must have on hand prior to placing an esophageal obturator airway. Prior to placement, the EMT-Intermediate must assure that the airway is clear of obstruction (suction) and the patient is pre-oxygenated (oxygen source and oropharyngeal airway) with a bag-valve-mask. Also, lubrication ensures a smoother attempt at proper placement with less chance of esophageal trauma. A stylet and laryngoscope are not items that are utilized in the placement of the esophageal obturator airway. *(1.7.25)*

34.

D. The pilot balloon serves as a visible indicator of the hidden inflatable tracheal cuff. If the pilot balloon will not remain inflated, the EMT-Intermediate must immediately suspect a problem with the inflatable cuff. In this situation, the endotracheal tube should be removed and the patient reintubated with another tube. The bag-valve-mask connects to the 15/22 mm adapter at the proximal end of the tube, not the pilot balloon. *(1.7.28)*

35.

D. Visualization of the endotracheal tube passing between the vocal cords is the greatest assurance of proper tube placement. *(1.7.33)*

36.

C. An unsecured endotracheal tube can slide down inside the trachea stimulating parasympathetic receptors located near and on the carina. Once activated, these receptors can precipitate bradycardia and hypotension. Securing an endotracheal tube does little in terms of preventing a patient from biting down on the tube. A bite block or oropharyngeal airway would better serve to accomplish this task. Also, the metal stylet should be immediately removed once the tube has passed between the vocal cords. Because the pilot balloon is located outside the patient's mouth at the proximal end of the endotracheal tube, securing the tube has little to so with the unlikely event of rupture. *(1.7.33)*

37.

C. The normal range for arterial $PaCO_2$ is 35 to 45 mmHg. *(1.7.4)*

38.

D. Hypercapnia in a healthy individual will cause the respiratory activity to increase. This increase in rate and depth, known as hyperventilation, allows more $PaCO_2$ to be exhaled until it is lowered to normal. *(1.7.5)*

39.

A. Hypocapnia does not stimulate the central and peripheral chemoreceptors, thus a decrease in $PaCO_2$ has no immediate effect on the respiratory activity of a healthy individual. The respiratory rate and depth will remain essentially unchanged. The $PaCO_2$ accumulates, gradually returning to normal levels. *(1.7.6)*

40.

B. Possible causes of increased CO_2 production include any activities that result in increased metabolic activity, like fever and shivering. Asthma, respiratory depression due to drug overdose, head injury, airway obstruction, or paralysis of the respiratory muscles all may contribute to the decreased elimination of CO_2 resulting in respiratory acidosis. *(1.7.7)*

41.

A. An esophageal obturator airway should be removed only if the patient becomes fully conscious or if tracheal intubation has been performed. *(1.7.16)*

42.

C. Because of the risk of esophageal injury, an esophageal obturator airway should only be used by trained personnel. An esophageal obturator airway is an alternative to endotracheal intubation because visualization is not required for insertion which can be accomplished without hyperextension of the neck. The esophageal obturator airway prevents gastric distention and regurgitation by obstructing the esophagus. *(1.7.17)*

43.

B. An oropharyngeal airway is an effective airway adjunct because it allows for air passage around and through the device and it prevents the tongue from obstructing the airway. However, among its disadvantages are failure to isolate the trachea, inflexibility, and that its insertion may stimulate vomiting. *(1.7.18)*

44.

C. When inserting an esophageal obturator airway, you should first hyperventilate the patient and then flex the patient's head slightly forward to prevent accidental tracheal intubation. *(1.7.26)*

45.

B. A relative contraindication for endotracheal intubation is major facial and neck trauma which may prevent recognition of landmarks. *(1.7.29)*

46.

C. Soft tissue injury is a complication associated with suctioning. Others include hypoxia and vagal stimulation. *(1.7.34)*

47.

A. The true vocal cords regulate the amount of air that passes through the larynx, as well as produce sound. The epiglottis is a leaf-shaped flap that prevents substances from entering the trachea while swallowing. Arytenoid folds are cupped tissues found posterior to the vocal cords and the lesser cornu are found superior to the hyoid bone. *(1.7.2a)*

48.

B. The esophagus lies directly behind the cricoid cartilage which forms a complete cartilaginous ring. The upper portion of the thyroid cartilage is attached to the hyoid bone. The vallecula is located above the epiglottis and the epiglottis is a leaf-shaped flap that is anterior to the pharynx. *(1.7.2b)*

49.

B. The epiglottis prevents food and drink from being aspirated into the glottis and trachea. The esophagus is positioned posterior to the larynx, the trachea is anterior to the esophagus and can be felt by palpating the neck. The trachea is supported by cartilage structures not the esophagus. *(1.7.2b)*

50.

B. The epiglottis protects the airway by closing off the trachea when food is being swallowed. The posterior portion of the thyroid cartilage is open and consists of muscle. Because the cricoid cartilage is a complete cartilaginous ring, when it is pressed during the Sellick's maneuver it compresses the esophagus, thus closing it. Tracheal cartilage are the incomplete rings that extend from the larynx to the bronchi. *(1.7.2c)*

51.

D. The epiglottis must be lifted to visualize the glottic opening. The vocal cords are hidden behind the epiglottis and cannot be visualized until the epiglottis is lifted. The hyoid bone is located below the chin but above the pharynx and is unique in the fact that it is the only bone that does not articulate with another bone, it is suspended by ligaments. The vocal folds are a point of attachment for the arytenoid cartilage and does not effect visualization of the glottic opening. *(1.7.2c)*

52.

A. The most common airway obstruction is the tongue blocking the airway. This occurs when the relaxed tongue falls back against the rear of the pharynx occluding the airway. *(1.7.2d)*

53.

C. The submandibular (below the mandible or lower jaw) muscle provides direct support of the tongue and indirect support of the epiglottis. Poor muscle tone of this muscle may lead to an obstructed airway. *(1.7.2d)*

54.

D. The true vocal cords, which are pale or pearly white, are the structures in the glottic opening that are easiest to identify. The tracheal cartilage is found in the trachea and gives the trachea its structural form. Aryepiglottic folds are landmarks that help to identify the glottic area but do not border the glottis. The false vocal cords lie above the true vocal cords. *(1.7.2e)*

55.

A. Because of its size and structure, the rigid catheter, or tonsil tip, should only be used when suctioning the upper airway. Vigorous insertion can cause lacerations and bleeding. *(1.7.9)*

56.

B. Suctioning water between each suctioning attempt will clear the tubing, as well as lubricate the catheter. The suction cannot be reversed; this would be dangerous for it would spread secretions. Never use a petroleum lubricant near the airway or rubber tubing. Replacing the tubing would be costly and wasteful, but be prepared to replace it if needed. *(1.7.10)*

57.

A. The correct way to measure the length needed to suction the mouth and oropharynx is from the corner of the mouth to the tip of the ear. When suctioning the nose and nasopharynx, the length is determined by measuring the catheter from the tip of the patient's nose to their ear. *(1.7.10)*

58.

A. The battery-powered suction unit becomes totally ineffective once the battery runs out. This suction unit can be operated by one rescuer. The suction can and should be reduced when suctioning infants and children and the unit is manufactured as a portable. *(1.7.11)*

59.

D. The hand-powered unit is the most effective when suctioning thick, tenacious substances. The hand-powered unit also does not require a power source other than that of the EMT-I. This reduces the maintenance costs and the threat of failure caused by a failed power source. *(1.7.11)*

60.

D. The rigid suction catheter is not used to suction the laryngopharynx and glottic space. This area of the airway is below the epiglottis and is too far down the airway to effectively suction with the rigid catheter. *(1.7.12)*

61.

D. The distal cuff when inflated with 30 to 35 cc of air from a syringe will block off the esophagus and prevent the regurgitation of stomach contents, thus protecting the airway. The esophageal obturator airway does not block the trachea. The inflated mask seal blocks the escaping air from being lost between the mask and the face of the patient. Finally, the distal cuff does not secure the tube. *(1.7.24)*

62.

D. When preparing to insert the esophageal obturator airway, you should have the following equipment: esophageal obturator airway complete with mask and esophageal tube, 35-cc syringe for inflating the distal cuff, water-soluble lubricant to lubricate the bottom two thirds of the tube, suction unit that is ready for use to clear the airway, and stethoscope to check for proper placement of the tube. *(1.7.25)*

63.

A. A bag-valve-mask with a pop-off valve that cannot be disabled may lead to inadequate ventilations in some patients. A self-refilling bag is desired so there is no need for the oxygen pressure to refill the bag. The transparent mask will permit you to visualize if the patient vomits. The oxygen reservoir will allow you to deliver a high concentration of oxygen rather than the 21 percent that is found in the air. *(1.7.28)*

64.

A. An unresponsive patient that will not tolerate an oropharyngeal airway will not tolerate orotracheal intubation. A patient that does not respond to any type of stimulation is a high risk for aspiration and should be intubated. The trauma patient with copious amounts of blood in the airway needs to be suctioned and then intubated to prevent the aspiration of the blood. Do not intubate this patient by hyperextending the head. *(1.7.29)*

65.

C. If at any time you are unsure that the tube is properly placed, quickly remove the tube and use an alternative method such as an oropharyngeal airway and a bag-valve-mask to ventilate the patient. If the tube is left in the esophagus, the patient will die. The patient must be ventilated with the bag-valve-mask prior to re-intubating, or severe hypoxia will result. Remember, if you see the tube pass through the vocal cords, you are in the correct place. *(1.7.30)*

66.

D. Bradycardia caused by stimulating the back of the throat may occur when suctioning the mouth and oropharynx, not down the endotracheal tube. *(1.7.34)*

67.

D. The epiglottis, gag reflex nerves, and vallecula are located in the pharynx. The vocal cords are found in the larynx. *(1.7.1)*

68.

C. Narcotics depress respiratory function, which results in decreased elimination of carbon dioxide. When $PaCO_2$ levels increase, pH levels decrease. The result of decreased pH is acidosis. In this case, the cause of the acidosis is a respiratory problem, consequently, the condition is a respiratory acidosis. *(1.7.5)*

69.

B. When carbon dioxide levels are increased hyperventilation occurs. Chemoreceptor stimulation increases, respiratory activity increases, resulting in more exhaled CO_2 and eventually a return to normal $PaCO_2$ levels. *(1.7.6)*

70.

C. Fever, muscle exertion, shivering, and metabolic processes all result in the increased production of carbon dioxide. Airway obstruction, narcotic drugs, obstructive disease states, and impairment of respiratory muscles are all causes of increased CO_2 retention. *(1.7.7)*

71.

A. Respiratory alkalosis is caused by hyperventilation and causing the elimination of carbon dioxide. This results in the loss of hydrogen ions and an elevated pH. *(1.7.8)*

72.

C. The esophageal obturator airway prevents gastric distention and regurgitation by blocking the passageway from the stomach to the hypopharynx. The esophageal obturator airway requires the patient to be unresponsive with an absent gag reflex. It delivers ventilation at the level of the hypopharynx only, therefore, it cannot guarantee a direct route to the respiratory passages. *(1.7.17)*

73.

C. The endotracheal tube isolates the trachea, which allows complete control of the airway. It also offers a direct route to the respiratory passages, thereby allowing for easy suctioning and medication administration. *(1.7.18)*

74.

D. The absence of breath sounds and chest rise are indicative of placement of the tube in the trachea, particularly if sounds are present over the epigastrium.

The esophageal obturator airway should be removed and another attempt made. *(1.7.27)*

75.

D. Intubating the pediatric patient requires a straight laryngoscope blade, as the epiglottis is floppy, so it needs to be lifted directly. The narrowest part of the pediatric airway is the cricoid cartilage. When an appropriately sized endotracheal tube is inserted, a seal is created at the cricoid level. The cricoid ring serves as a functional cuff. *(1.7.28)*

76.

A. The esophageal gastric tube airway, pharyngeal lumen airway, and the esophageal tracheal combitube airway are acceptable alternative airway adjuncts for the apneic patient. Intubation of the trachea, when possible, is the preferred technique for managing the airway. *(1.7.30)*

77.

B. The epiglottis is located within the laryngopharynx and is superior to the larynx. *(1.7.2c)*

78.

A. The tongue is located anterior and superior to the larynx. *(1.7.2d)*

79.

A. The anterior portion of the larynx is known as the thyroid cartilage. It is commonly called the Adam's apple. The cricoid cartilage forms the inferior border of the larynx, which makes up the first tracheal ring. *(1.7.2d)*

80.

B. The false vocal cords are located lateral to the true vocal cords. The true vocal cords regulate air entering the larynx. As the muscles of the larynx contract the vocal cords change shape and vibrate. This change in shape coupled with the movement of air across the vocal cords produces sound. Passage of an endotracheal tube between the true vocal cords prevents the creation of sound or the production of a cough. *(1.7.2e)*

81.

D. The space between the vocal cords is known as the glottis or the glottic opening. The vallecula is the junction of the tongue and the epiglottis. The pyriform fossa is located on both sides of the epiglottis. *(1.7.2e)*

82.

C. The larynx is located inferior to the pharynx. The lower-most portion of the pharynx is known as the hypopharynx or the laryngopharynx. *(1.7.2f)*

83.

C. The most superior region of the pharynx is called the nasopharynx. The oropharynx and the laryngopharynx are the other functional subdivisions. *(1.7.2f)*

84.

D. The normal PaO_2 in the body is 80 to 100 mmHg. Atmospheric air pressure (at sea level) is equivalent to 760 mmHg and the PaO_2 or $PaCO_2$ refers to the "partial pressure" of oxygen or carbon dioxide in the body. This is calculated as a percent of the total volume of gases present in normal atmospheric air. *(1.7.3)*

85.

D. A mouth powered suction device is not available for adult patients. However, one is available for use in neonatal patients. It is called a DeLee suction trap. All others are common sources of suction for suction units. *(1.7.11)*

86.

B. The whistle tip and the tonsil tip are the most commonly used catheters in prehospital care. The tonsil tip is also called the Yankauer. *(1.7.12)*

87.

C. The whistle-tip or soft suction catheter is a long flexible tube. It is smaller in diameter than the tonsil tip suction catheter and for this reason it is not well suited to the removal of large amounts of fluids or blood. The whistle tip is used for deep tracheal suctioning. The tonsil tip is used for the removal of large amounts of blood or secretions in the oropharynx. *(1.7.12)*

88.

C. For large amounts of fluid or vomit, use a Yankauer or tonsil-tip suction catheter. The distal opening is much larger than a whistle-tip suction catheter and better able to handle large volumes and larger particulate matter. *(1.7.13)*

89.

A. A whistle-tip or soft suction catheter is thin, flexible, and long enough to provide tracheal suctioning. The whistle-tip catheter may be placed through the external nares, oropharynx, through a oropharyngeal airway or into an endotracheal tube. *(1.7.13)*

90.

D. If airway patentcy cannot be achieved with an endotracheal tube, an ETC airway is acceptable in the trauma patient. An ETC airway should not be attempted in the patient with an intact gag reflex, excessive bleeding in the oropharynx, or if caustic poison has been ingested. *(1.7.14)*

91.

D. A stylet is used to assist with placement of an endotracheal tube. It is not required for ETC airway placement. An assembled esophageal obturator airway complete with mask and tube, suction unit, syringe, lubricant, and stethoscope should also be prepared. *(1.7.25)*

92.

A. The correct sequence for insertion of the esophageal obturator airway is hyperventilate, prepare equipment, lubricate tube, place head in a neutral position, elevate tongue and mandible, insert tube, seal mask against face, ventilate, confirm tube placement, inflate the cuff, and continue ventilation of the patient. *(1.7.26)*

93.

D. Ventilate the patient and check for proper tube placement prior to inflation of the distal balloon. You must ensure that the tube is properly positioned in the esophagus and not in the trachea before inflation. Improper placement in the trachea will result in the patient not being ventilated. The head is placed in a neutral position, not flexed or extended. *(1.7.26)*

94.

D. The most common cause of inadequate ventilation and oxygenation is the failure to provide an adequate mask to face seal. It is difficult to maintain an adequate seal. Two rescuers should ideally perform ventilation, one holding the mask seal with two hands and the other squeezing the bag-valve-mask. *(1.7.27)*

95.

A. All of the items are contraindications for the use of the esophageal obturator airway except for a patient who is 16 years of age. The device is contraindicated in patient younger than 16 years of age. *(1.7.29)*

96.

D. The best choice would be to use your fingers to digitally intubate the patient. Nasotracheal intubation is difficult to accomplish in a non-breathing patient. Orotracheal intubation would be difficult given the patient's position. Head movement that may occur during placement would also make this method difficult. The use of the lighted stylet in direct sunlight is not practical. *(1.7.30)*

97.

C. Airway management skills such as endotracheal intubation are psychomotor skills. You must practice these skills constantly to maintain your proficiency. Reading, watching, and listening will not take the place of actually performing or practicing the skill. *(1.7.31)*

98.

A. Endotracheal intubation must be accomplished in less than 30 seconds. After 30 seconds, ventilate the patient for 2 minutes prior to attempting the intubation again. Try holding your breath from the time you stop ventilations until you need a breath. If you need a breath you can be sure the patient does as well. *(1.7.32)*

99.

A. Carbon dioxide levels in the blood stream are a direct reflection of alveolar ventilation. As such, any increase in the patient's minute ventilation will cause a lowering of the $PaCO_2$ value. Oxygen levels move opposite of carbon dioxide levels, but are not dependant upon it. The extra acid produced from the heightened muscular respiratory effort will be buffered by the body's normal mechanisms. *(1.7.8)*

100.

B. An infant with an airway occlusion needs suctioning just as much as an adult patient, and there are no dangers of inherent hypoxemia as long as the skill is done correctly. You should not suction longer than 5 to 10 seconds to avoid hypoxemia, and should only suction while withdrawing the catheter. *(1.7.9)*

101.

D. Portable suction units can be used with either a tonsil-tip catheter or whistle-tip catheter. Most units will have two levels of suctioning so that you can decrease the suctioning strength with the French tip. Always clean and disinfect all equipment and be sure to assemble it correctly and charge the batteries so it will be functional the next time it is needed. *(1.7.10)*

102.

D. Utilization of the EOA is not without its limitations. Even when properly placed, the patient may still aspirate vomitus or blood in the upper airway. Additionally, if the cuff deflates, the device will become less effective. And with aggressive insertion, mucosal damage with resultant hemorrhage may occur. *(1.7.23)*

103.

B. Directly posterior to the tongue is the oropharynx, and when the unconscious patient becomes supine, gravity causes the tongue to relax backwards and block the airway. The nasopharynx is located superior to the oropharynx, and the hypopharynx (also known as laryngopharynx) is located inferior to the oropharynx. *(1.7.1)*

104.

C. A stylet is an adjunctive piece of equipment needed for intubation when the glottic opening is located anterior or cephalad. The syringe is needed to inflate the tracheal cuff, the blade (#3 or #4 for an adult) is necessary for visualization, and the laryngoscope handle is necessary and interfaces with the laryngoscope blade. *(1.7.28)*

105.

D. Although all are necessary components of a comprehensive continuing education program, doing return demonstrations of a skill would best provide the opportunity for the EMT-I to stay efficient with the skill. Reading, listening, and watching will reinforce only the cognitive aspect of the skill. *(1.7.31)*

106.

A. Insertion of an endotracheal tube is very important so that it is not advanced too far. To assure proper placement, insert the tube until the proximal side of the cuff passes just beyond the true vocal cords, through the glottic opening. *(1.7.2e)*

107.

B. The larynx, comprised of the thyroid, cricoid and epiglottis cartilage, houses the vocal cords. The pharynx, commonly known as the throat, lies superior to the larynx and is a passage way for both food and air. *(1.7.2f)*

108.

D. In a healthy adult the normal PaO_2 is 80 to 100 mmHg. Any value below 80 mmHg is considered abnormal and is a common finding with hypoxemia. *(1.7.3)*

109.

A. In a healthy adult the normal $PaCO_2$ is 35 to 45 mmHg. Any value below 35 mmHg is considered to be respiratory alkalosis, and values over 45 mmHg are termed respiratory acidosis. *(1.7.4)*

110.

B. There are numerous contraindications for EOA placement, one of these is ingestion of a caustic substance since the EOA tube may then perforate the injured esophageal walls. There are height restrictions, although 5¢11≤ is acceptable, and gastric ulcers have no bearing since the tube does not reach the stomach when properly placed. Absence of a gag reflex is required for insertion as well. *(1.7.18)*

111.

D. All of the listed airways can still allow for aspirations since proper placement may find the tip of the long tube in the esophagus. The only airway adjunct that will guarantee a secure patient airway when properly placed is an endotracheal tube. *(1.7.23)*

112.

D. When providing tracheal suctioning, use a french catheter and a negative vacuum pressure of 80 to 120 mmHg. Pharyngeal or oral suctioning is usually greater than 120 mmHg. This skill could be completed by the EMT-I who intubated the patient, but suctioning time should still be limited to 5 to 10 seconds to avoid undue hypoxemia. *(1.7.34)*

113.

B. The major advantage of an EOA over an OPA is that the EOA will occlude the esophagus, thereby reducing the likelihood of regurgitation and aspiration of vomitus. If the patient is bleeding above the cuff however, neither the EOA nor OPA can prevent aspiration. And as a reminder, neither device can be inserted with an intact gag reflex. *(1.7.14)*

114.

B. Insertion of the EOA is a blind technique, which means you do not need to visualize any airway structures. This is considered to be a benefit of the device. You must still implement a manual airway technique to ensure an airway and if the mask is not firmly placed on the face, an air leak will occur which renders the device useless. *(1.7.15)*

115.

C. If the patient's level of consciousness improves to the point that the device cannot be tolerated due to the gag reflex, it must be removed. Otherwise, spontaneous breathing, no vomiting, and arrival at the ED does not mean the patient no longer needs airway maintenance, and the EOA is left in place. *(1.7.16)*

116.

B. The series of perforated holes on the proximal 1/3 of the cuff are to allow the positive pressure ventilation to enter the trachea and exhaled air to exit. Remember the ventilation device fits over the outside end of the tube and the esophageal end of the tube is blocked off (isolating the stomach). There is a suctioning port, but it is located on the mask. *(1.7.24)*

117.

A. The vocal cords are housed and protected by the thyroid cartilage that is part of the larynx, along with the carina and epiglottis. The trachea is inferior to the larynx, and the hyoid bone is embedded in the submandibular muscles superior to the larynx. *(1.7.2a)*

118.

A. If an endotracheal tube becomes misplaced there will be abdominal distention that may become severe. The presence of moisture in the ET tube is expected, and a decrease in bagging resistance is not characteristic of a misplaced tube, in fact it should increase if misplaced. Finally, high CO_2 levels are expected with appropriate tube placement. *(1.7.33)*

119.

C. The trachea bifurcates into the right and left mainstem bronchus at the anatomic location called the carina. *(1.7.1)*

120.

B. The tube will first pass through the oropharynx, the hypopharynx, the glottic opening, then between the vocal cords in the larynx and into the trachea. *(1.7.2)*

121.

D. The esophagus is located posterior to the glottic opening in the hypopharynx. The glottic opening and esophagus are both located in the hypopharynx. *(1.7.2b)*

122.

A. The larynx begins to spasm, causing the vocal cords to close when water, food, or other substances enter the glottic opening. This protective reflex causes the patient to choke forcefully and perceive a feeling of not being able to catch his/her breath. *(1.7.2c)*

123.

B. Both the esophagus and opening to the larynx, the glottic opening, are located in the lower portion of the pharnx. *(1.7.2f)*

124.

A. The patient is experiencing hyperventilation syndrome in which he is breathing fast and deep. His elevated respiratory rate and increased tidal volume will cause him to take in excessive amounts of oxygen and blow off significant amounts of carbon dioxide resulting in an elevated PaO_2 level exceeding 100 mmHg and a decreased $PaCO_2$ below 40 mmHg. *(1.7.3)*

125.

C. You would expect the PaO_2 level to be greater than 100 mmHg and the $PaCO_2$ level to be less than 35 mmHg. When hyperventilating a patient, your goal is to increase the PaO_2 and decrease the $PaCO_2$ levels. *(1.7.4)*

126.

B. As the $PaCO_2$ level rises the pH value will begin to drop below the normal 7.40 and the respiratory rate and depth will increase to blow off carbon dioxide. By removing carbon dioxide, the amount of carbonic acid is reduced and the blood becomes less acidic causing the pH value to rise. *(1.7.5)*

127.

A. The chemoreceptors constantly measure the $PaCO_2$, PaO_2, and pH levels in the blood. When the $PaCO_2$ level rises, the pH value decreases, or the PaO_2 level decreases, the respiratory system increases the rate and depth of respiration to decrease the amount of CO_2, which in turn decreases the amount of carbonic acid. *(1.7.6)*

128.

C. The patient is hypoventilating due to a possible head injury. The inadequate ventilation will cause the PaO_2 level to drop less than 90 mmHg and the $PaCO_2$ level to rise above 45 mmHg as CO_2 is retained. *(1.7.7)*

129.

D. In order to decrease the $PaCO_2$ level it is necessary to reduce the carbon dioxide concentration in the arterial blood. This can be achieved by removing more CO_2 from the alveoli through hyperventila-

tion of the patient. During hyperventilation, less CO_2 is in the alveoli, therefore, more CO_2 can move from the capillary into the alveoli to be exhaled off. *(1.7.8)*

130.

B. The priority is to clear the airway with suction then to perform a manual maneuver to open the airway. Once the airway is opened, it is necessary to assess and manage the ventilation before checking the pulse. *(1.7.9)*

131.

D. It is necessary to suction the nasopharynx. An oropharyngeal airway will not protect the trachea from aspiration of vomitus or other substances. If the nasopharynx is not cleared, the vomitus will likely be aspirated into the trachea with the first few ventilations. *(1.7.13)*

132.

A. The main purpose of the esophageal obturator airway (EOA) is to reduce the incidence of regurgitation of vomitus. The EOA is not a means to ventilate a patient, but an airway adjunct. Also, it is associated with operator fatigue leading to poor mask seal and ineffective tidal volume. *(1.7.14)*

133.

B. Esophageal varices is a disease process in which the esophageal veins dilate and rupture. This condition is associated with massive bleeding in the esophagus. The patient frequently will swallow the blood which irritates the stomach causing regurgitation. Airway management is usually very challenging in these patients. The best method to manage this patient is to place him on his side to facilitate drainage of blood from the airway, suction, and begin bag-valve-mask ventilation. An EOA is contraindicated in esophageal disease. In addition, it will not prevent aspiration of contents coming from the upper airway or proximal portion of the esophagus. *(1.7.15)*

134.

C. The major disadvantage of the EOA is that a good mask seal must be maintained along with a head tilt–chin lift or jaw thrust maneuver. This commonly leads to operator fatigue, poor mask seal and subsequent inadequate ventilation. *(1.7.23)*

135.

B. The most common problem associated with the EOA is inadequate ventilation resulting from a poor mask seal. *(1.7.27)*

136.

C. One disadvantage of endotracheal intubation is the need for training and skill in performing a laryngoscopy, and knowledge of upper airway anatomy in order to successfully place an endotracheal tube. Other devices like the ETC do not require visualization, much skill, or a significant amount of training. *(1.7.29)*

137.

D. It is necessary to immediately intubate this patient to control the airway and prevent aspiration of blood. An oropharyngeal airway or an EOA will not prevent aspiration of blood coming from the face or upper airway. The patient cannot be placed in a lateral recumbent position due to the suspicion of a spinal injury and the need to perform manual in-line spinal stabilization. *(1.7.32)*

138.

A. Endotracheal intubation requires continuous skill maintenance and knowledge of the upper airway anatomy. The most preferred method of intubation is the orotracheal route using the laryngoscope and direct visualization. Endotracheal intubation can be successfully performed by many allied health personnel, inlcuding EMT-Paramedics, EMT-Intermediates, and EMT-Basics. Endotracheal intubation can be performed on a variety of patients who require airway control, not just patients in cardiac arrest. *(1.7.31)*

139.

C. The best method to check placement of the endotracheal tube is to perform a laryngoscopy and visually inspect the tube placement through the glottic opening. *(1.7.33)*

8 Assessment and Management of Shock

chapter objectives

Questions in this chapter relate to DOT objectives 1.8.1–1.8.37. Please see the Appendix for more information.

1. The primary role of intravascular proteins is to maintain:
   A. hydrostatic pressure.
   B. colloid osmotic pressure.
   C. intracellular pressure.
   D. interstitial pressure.

2. For which of the following patients would a hypertonic intravenous solution be most appropriate?
   A. a dehydrated patient
   B. a congestive heart failure patient
   C. a burn patient
   D. a hypovolemic patient

3. Which of the following molecules requires active transport to move it across the cellular membranes?
   A. albumin
   B. calcium
   C. glucose
   D. water

4. A patient with an increase in metabolic activity will attempt to buffer the increased acid load by initially:
   A. increasing the respiratory rate.
   B. creating more carbonic acid.
   C. increasing renal excretion of hydrogen ions.
   D. decreasing the circulating bicarbonate levels.

5. Which of the following will most likely cause respiratory acidosis?
   A. an increase in the respiratory rate and a decrease in the respiratory depth
   B. a decrease in the respiratory rate and an increase in the respiratory depth
   C. a decrease in the respiratory rate and a decrease in the respiratory depth
   D. an increase in the respiratory rate and an increase in the respiratory depth

6. A drop in cardiac output from volume loss would initially be detected by:
   A. chemoreceptors.
   B. baroreceptors.
   C. pressoreceptors.
   D. adenoreceptors.

7. Which of the following contributes most to diminished coronary artery perfusion in hypovolemic shock states?
   A. diminished preload
   B. shortened diastole
   C. increased systemic vascular resistance
   D. increased glomerular filtration

8. You are treating a 37-year-old male who was struck by an automobile while jogging. Your partner estimates that the patient lost a significant amount of blood, but you note that there is still a radial pulse present. This finding means:
   A. the cardiovascular system is still able to perfuse distal extremities.
   B. the patient has not really lost very much blood.
   C. the heart is not compromised.
   D. the arterial oxygen saturation is still adequate.

9. The movement of oxygen from the alveoli to the red blood cell occurs:
   A. by active transport.
   B. down the pressure gradient.

C. by facilitated transport.

D. by osmosis.

10. What negative feedback mechanism will become activated to maintain blood pressure when circulating volume is lost?

A. precapillary spinchters close

B. arterio-venule shunts close

C. precapillary spinchters relax

D. postcapillary spinchters relax

11. A patient was attacked and stabbed several times in the chest. A drop in pulmonary perfusion occurs as a result of the injuries. Which of the following is most likely the cause?

A. an increase in arterial tone

B. venous vasospasms

C. a lengthened diastole

D. a drop in stroke volume

12. Administering an isotonic crystalloid solution intravenously to a hypovolemic patient will increase of cardiac output primarily by increasing:

A. preload.

B. heart rate.

C. contractility.

D. afterload.

13. You have been administering a large amount of isotonic crystalloid solution to a trauma patient. After a period of time, you notice slight jugular venous distention and bilateral crackles upon auscultation of the lungs. You should:

A. change over to a hypotonic solution and continue fluid administration.

B. disconnect the IV since there is volume overload.

C. slow the IV infusion rate and consult medical control.

D. leave the infusion running at the current rate and consult medical control.

14. Which of the following IV solution/equipment setups is most appropriate for a volume-depleted patient?

A. 0.9% NaCl, 16-gauge angio, macrodrip administration set

B. 5% dextrose in water, 20-gauge angio, minidrip administration set

C. 0.45% NaCl, 14-gauge angio, macrodrip administration set

D. lactated Ringer's, 14-gauge angio, microdrip administration set

15. A 45-year-old man was stabbed with an ice pick that penetrated the heart. The patient is presenting with severe dyspnea and pulmonary edema. Which heart valve is most likely affected by this injury?

A. pulmonic valve

B. mitral valve

C. tricuspid valve

D. aortic valve

16. An increase in the force of contraction of the myocardium will cause:

A. an increase in the heart rate.

B. a decrease in afterload.

C. increase in blood pressure.

D. none of the above.

17. You are treating a patient with hypotension and severe dyspnea. Which of the following assessment findings would be most consistent with dyspnea caused by a left ventricular failure?

A. acute excessive peripheral edema

B. decreased breath sounds

C. jugular venous distention

D. rales upon auscultation

18. You are treating a multi-system trauma patient who is in cardiac arrest. All of the following treatment considerations for this patient are correct, **except**:

    A. you should avoid intubation since hypoxemia is probably severe.

    B. you should provide full spinal immobilization prior to transport.

    C. you should utilize the AED if medical control allows.

    D. you should initiate an IV of normal saline or ringers lactate.

19. You are assessing a hypotensive, anxious, tachycardic patient who was struck with a baseball bat in the upper-left quadrant of the abdomen. Which of the following is a first priority in treatment for this patient?

    A. oxygen administration

    B. fluid replacement

    C. full spinal immobilization

    D. drug administration

20. The best estimate of systemic vascular resistance is provided by the:

    A. pulse pressure.

    B. diastolic pressure.

    C. presence of a radial pulse.

    D. systolic pressure.

21. Which of the following statements best describes the role of sodium?

    A. regulates water distribution

    B. chief intracellular ion

    C. used as fuel by the cells

    D. responsible for metabolism

22. The intracellular concentration of potassium is ten times the concentration of extracellular potassium. The cellular membrane is relatively impermeable to potassium. Based on osmosis, which of the following statements is most correct?

    A. Water will move out of the cell.

    B. Potassium will move out of the cell.

    C. No change will occur.

    D. Water will move into the cell.

23. What process is responsible for the movement of oxygen molecules from the arterial blood into the intracellular space?

    A. diffusion

    B. active transport

    C. osmosis

    D. saturation

24. Which of the following structures is primarily responsible for maintaining concentrations of sodium?

    A. vasomotor center

    B. kidney

    C. liver

    D. lungs

25. An individual's $PaCO_2$ is 31 mmHg. Which of the following conditions would you expect would correlate with this reading?

    A. decrease in pH

    B. increase in CO_2

    C. decrease in saturated hemoglobin

    D. increase in pH

26. A woman informs you that her grandfather has been vomiting heavily for the past 3 days. In addition, the patient has had a decreased level of consciousness and intermittent convulsions. You suspect this individual is suffering from:

    A. respiratory alkalosis.

    B. metabolic acidosis.

    C. hypervolemia.

    D. metabolic alkalosis.

27. Baroreceptor reflexes cause a change primarily in which of these components of the cardiovascular system?

A. vena cava

B. venules

C. arterioles

D. capillaries

28. A 17-year-old female has fallen down 14 stairs. In your assessment, you note a large laceration to the posterior head and some deformity to the left tibia. Vitals include: BP 88/68, HR 112/regular, RR 24/shallow. The best treatment for this patient prior to transport would include:

    A. begin BVM ventilation and immobilize to a backboard

    B. place patient in a semi-Fowler's position and begin BVM ventilation

    C. apply a traction splint to the left tibia, begin BVM ventilation

    D. apply the PASG and a non-rebreather at 15 lpm

29. You are managing a patient in hemorrhagic shock from a gunshot wound to the chest. After administering 2 liters of lactated Ringer's, the patient regains a radial pulse with a blood pressure of 118/86. You should:

    A. continue rapid transport and keep IVs wide open.

    B. back down to a nonemergent transport and set the administration of lactated Ringer's at TKO.

    C. continue rapid transport and set administration of lactated Ringer's at TKO.

    D. begin nonemergent transport and consider the administration of plasma.

30. The best indicator of effective fluid therapy in a hypovolemic patient is:

    A. presence of diaphoresis.

    B. regain radial pulse.

C. warm skin.

D. increased blood pressure.

31. The greatest limiting factor to the rate of fluid replacement is:

    A. lumen of the catheter.

    B. size of the vein.

    C. type of crystalloid.

    D. size of the fluid bag.

32. The first step in glucose metabolism results in the formation of pyruvic acid. This is a(n):

    A. lactate process.

    B. anaerobic process.

    C. aerobic process.

    D. gluconeogenic process.

33. The administration of oxygen and ventilatory support are critical to the management of shock by reducing:

    A. acidosis and blood loss.

    B. blood loss and respiratory effort.

    C. respiratory effort and hypoxia.

    D. hypoxia and acidosis.

34. Hypovolemia impacts cardiac output by:

    A. reducing preload, thus decreasing cardiac output.

    B. increasing afterload, thus increasing cardiac output.

    C. reducing afterload, thus decreasing cardiac output.

    D. increasing preload, thus increasing cardiac output.

35. Interstitial fluid includes all of the following, **except**:

    A. aqueous humor.

    B. plasma.

    C. cerebrospinal fluid.

    D. lymph.

36. A protein which plays a critical transport role in the body is:
    A. hemoglobin.
    B. interleukin.
    C. collagen.
    D. lipase.

37. Administration of a hypotonic solution will cause:
    A. water to move out of red blood cells causing the cells to shrink.
    B. no significant change in the size of red blood cells.
    C. water to move into red blood cells causing the cells to swell.
    D. free movement of water into and out of red blood cells.

38. The sodium-potassium pump in myocardial cells is an example of:
    A. active transport.
    B. facilitated diffusion.
    C. osmosis.
    D. diffusion.

39. The dynamic relationship that reflects the relative concentration of hydrogen ions in the body is known as:
    A. metabolic acidosis.
    B. acid-base balance.
    C. metabolic alkalosis.
    D. bicarbonate buffer system.

40. Metabolic acidosis can result from:
    A. hyperventilation.
    B. prolonged vomiting.
    C. increased bicarbonate.
    D. diarrhea.

41. The body compensates for shock in all of the following ways, **except**:

A. vasoconstriction of the arterioles and venules of the skin.
B. initiation of the renin-angiotension pathway to increase blood pressure.
C. intravascular clotting maintains blood volume by limiting blood loss.
D. increased reabsorption of sodium and water to restore blood volume.

42. A disadvantage associated with the use of 5% dextrose in water for fluid replacement is:
    A. the glucose is quickly metabolized and leaves free water in the intravascular space.
    B. edema results from the retention of glucose in the intravascular space.
    C. glucose supplies more calories than are necessary for metabolism.
    D. alkalosis follows the administration of large volumes of glucose.

43. The flow rate for fluid replacement should be based on the:
    A. protocols or on-line medical control.
    B. patient's vital signs, mental status, and peripheral pulses.
    C. development of peripheral edema, and diastolic blood pressure.
    D. transport time and distance.

44. All of the following are disadvantages associated with the use of central lines for field fluid replacement, **except**:
    A. central venous cannulation requires the use of a sterile procedure.
    B. central lines usually require X-ray confirmation of placement.
    C. the predictable location of central veins permits rapid access.
    D. there is a higher complication rate associated with central lines.

45. Which of the following will reverse anaerobic metabolism?
    A. decrease perfusion and increase oxygenation
    B. increase perfusion state and decrease hypoxia
    C. increase perfusion and decrease oxygenation
    D. decrease perfusion state and increase hypoxia

46. When oxygen in the lungs leaves an area of higher concentration and enters an area of lower concentration in the pulmonary capillaries this process is called:
    A. diffusion.
    B. osmosis.
    C. active transport.
    D. facilitated transport.

47. Which of the following will improve cardiac output?
    A. an increase in stroke volume and an increase in heart rate
    B. a decrease in stroke volume and a decrease in heart rate
    C. increase in systemic vascular resistance
    D. a reduction in preload

48. Constriction of the venous side of the vascular system will result in:
    A. decreased cardiac preload.
    B. increased cardiac preload.
    C. decreased afterload.
    D. decreased blood pressure.

49. Which of the following compartments contains the highest percentage of total body water?
    A. intravascular
    B. interstitial
    C. extracellular
    D. intracellular

50. Which cation plays an important role in electrical impulse transmission and is the most prevalent cation in the intracellular fluid?
    A. Potassium (K^+)
    B. Calcium (Ca^{++})
    C. Sodium (Na^+)
    D. Magnesium (Mg^{++})

51. Certain molecules move across the cell membrane by facilitated diffusion. To accomplish this they need the assistance of:
    A. leukocytes.
    B. lipids.
    C. sodium.
    D. proteins.

52. When a solute moves across the cell membrane from an area of higher concentration to an area of lower concentration, without the use of energy, this is known as:
    A. diffusion.
    B. osmosis.
    C. active transport.
    D. facilitated diffusion.

53. The sodium-potassium pump is an example of:
    A. centrifugation.
    B. hypertonic diffusion.
    C. facilitated transport.
    D. active transport.

54. Which of the following is the most prevalent cation in the extracellular fluid and plays a major role in regulating water distribution?
    A. Sodium (NA^+)
    B. Potassium (K^+)
    C. Phosphate (HPO_4)
    D. Chloride (Cl^-)

55. From the selection below, which of the following represents an acidotic pH?

    A. 7.57

    B. 7.43

    C. 7.39

    D. 7.27

56. When the bicarbonate buffer system does not significantly alter the hydrogen ion concentration, the next system to intervene in an attempt to increase the pH of the body is:

    A. renal system.

    B. respiratory system.

    C. hepatic system.

    D. vascular system.

57. Your patient presents with bradypnea and hypopnea. The blood gases reveal elevations in the CO_2 level only. The patient is most likely suffering from:

    A. metabolic alkalosis.

    B. metabolic acidosis.

    C. respiratory alkalosis.

    D. respiratory acidosis.

58. Your patient is experiencing an anxiety episode and has been hyperventilating for some time. Your patient is likely to be experiencing:

    A. metabolic alkalosis.

    B. metabolic acidosis.

    C. respiratory alkalosis.

    D. respiratory acidosis.

59. Which of the following is a common cause of metabolic acidosis?

    A. prolonged hypoperfusion and hypoxia at the cellular level or serious infection

    B. hypoventilation and the retention of carbon dioxide increasing hydrogen ions

    C. too much bicarbonate ions from ingestion of excessive amounts of antacids

    D. hyperventilation that eliminates CO_2 resulting in the loss of hydrogen ions

60. Your patient has been vomiting for the past two days. The arterial blood gas results show a $PaCO_2$ of 40 mmHg, a pH of 7.5, and a HCO_3 of 30. Your patient is most likely suffering from:

    A. respiratory acidosis.

    B. respiratory alkalosis.

    C. metabolic acidosis.

    D. metabolic alkalosis.

61. Which of the following best describes the physiology of decompensated shock?

    A. pre-capillary sphincters relax, post-capillary sphincters remain closed, capillary pressure diminishes

    B. cardiac preload is reduced, heart rate and peripheral vascular resistance increases to maintain blood pressure and perfusion

    C. prolonged inadequate tissue perfusion results in cellular death; the result is the same even if perfusion and vital signs return

    D. the venous system constricts, reducing the vascular container size, blood is directed away from non-critical areas such as the skin

62. You are assessing the perfusion status of your patient. You feel a carotid pulse but not a femoral pulse. This would indicate which of the following?

    A. The diastolic blood pressure is approximately 60 mmHg.

    B. The diastolic blood pressure is approximately 70 mmHg.

    C. The systolic blood pressure is approximately 60 mmHg.

    D. The systolic blood pressure is approximately 70 mmHg.

63. You are treating an unresponsive patient who has been involved in a motor vehicle crash. He has pale, cool, clammy skin, a RR of 42 and shallow, and only a carotid pulse present. Identify the most appropriate treatment for this patient.
    A. supine position, oxygen via nonrebreather mask, IV via 22-gauge catheter, transport
    B. elevation of the legs, high flow oxygen, IV fluids via 14-gauge catheter, rapid transport
    C. fowler position, ventilation, IV fluids via 20-gauge catheter, rapid transport
    D. positive pressure ventilation, IV fluids via 14-gauge catheter, rapid transport

64. In which of the following scenarios would the pneumatic antishock garment be contraindicated?
    A. multiple lacerations to the lower extremities with active bleeding
    B. penetrating knife wounds to the lower legs and the abdomen
    C. presence of moist rales lung sounds and pink frothy sputum
    D. trauma patient with multiple fractures of the lower extremities

65. Which of the following IV solutions will draw water from the intracellular compartment and interstitial space into the intravascular space?
    A. 5% dextrose in water
    B. normal saline
    C. lactated Ringer's
    D. dextran 40

66. Which IV fluid is not compatible with whole blood?
    A. plasmanate
    B. normal saline

C. lactated Ringer's
D. 5% dextrose in water

67. While infusing IV fluids you reassess your patient and find that the patient has developed signs of tachypnea, crackles upon ascultation, and jugular venous distention. You recognize these as signs of:
    A. thrombophlebitis.
    B. air embolism.
    C. pyrogenic reaction.
    D. circulation overload.

68. Which of the following techniques can be used to check the patentcy of the IV?
    A. Lower the IV bag below the IV site, if blood enters the tubing, the IV is patent.
    B. Compress the bag firmly to force the fluid out, if the fluid drips, the IV is patent.
    C. Replace the constricting band on the arm, if the flow continues, the IV is patent.
    D. Lift the bag above the IV site, if the drip chamber stops flowing, the IV is patent.

69. Which of the following IV catheters provides the greatest volume flow rate?
    A. 20-gauge, 5-cm catheter
    B. 20-gauge, 15-cm catheter
    C. 14-gauge, 5-cm catheter
    D. 14-gauge, 15-cm catheter

70. Which IV site is the most ideal location in a cardiac arrest?
    A. upper thigh
    B. back of the hand
    C. internal jugular
    D. external jugular

71. The most prevalent cations of the body are:
    A. calcium, magnesium, potassium, sodium.
    B. calcium, chloride, potassium, sodium.
    C. chloride, magnesium, potassium, sodium.
    D. calcium, chloride, magnesium, potassium.

72. The movement of a solvent across a semi-permeable membrane from an area of lower solute concentration to an area of higher solute concentration is referred to as:
    A. diffusion.
    B. osmosis.
    C. active transport.
    D. facilitated diffusion.

73. The movement of solutes across the semi-permeable membrane from an area of higher concentration to an area of lower concentration is called:
    A. diffusion.
    B. osmosis.
    C. active transport.
    D. facilitated diffusion.

74. The chief extracellular ion of the body is:
    A. bicarbonate.
    B. calcium.
    C. potassium.
    D. sodium.

75. Which of the following helps control the body's pH by retaining or eliminating carbon dioxide?
    A. the acid-base system
    B. the bicarbonate buffer system
    C. the kidneys
    D. the respiratory system

76. Which of the following conditions is a result of excessive loss of hydrogen ions from the body?
    A. metabolic acidosis
    B. metabolic alkalosis
    C. respiratory acidosis
    D. respiratory alkalosis

77. Inadequate cellular oxygenation results in:
    A. aerobic metabolism.
    B. anaerobic metabolism.
    C. glycolysis.
    D. the Kreb's cycle.

78. The body responds to shock by improving cardiac output. This can occur by:
    A. decreasing heart rate and decreasing stroke volume.
    B. decreasing heart rate and increasing stroke volume.
    C. increasing heart rate and decreasing stroke volume.
    D. increasing heart rate and increasing stroke volume.

79. When the baroreceptors in the carotid bodies and the aortic arch detect a decrease in blood pressure, which of the following occurs?
    A. stimulation of the parasympathetic nervous system resulting in a decreased heart rate
    B. stimulation of the parasympathetic nervous system resulting in an increased heart rate
    C. stimulation of the sympathetic nervous system resulting in a decreased heart rate
    D. stimulation of the sympathetic nervous system resulting in an increased heart rate

80. Which stage of shock is characterized by a drop in blood pressure?

A. compensated shock

B. fatal shock

C. irreversible shock

D. decompensated shock

81. The ideal replacement fluid for a patient in hemorrhagic shock is:

A. 5% dextrose in water

B. lactated Ringer's or normal saline

C. plasmanate

D. whole blood

82. You are ordered to administer an IV of a crystalloid solution over 90 minutes at 45 drops per minute using a microdrip administration set. How many milliliters would you deliver to the patient?

A. 0.5 ml

B. 2 ml

C. 67.5 ml

D. 120 ml

83. You are treating a patient who has experienced considerable blood loss. Which of the following sites would be most appropriate for initiating intravenous therapy?

A. antecubital fossa

B. dorsum of the hand

C. internal jugular vein

D. ventral forearm

84. Which statement best describes shock and its relationship to the body's metabolic process?

A. Low perfusion results in anaerobic metabolism, which leads to excessive lactic acid production.

B. Low perfusion results in aerobic metabolism, which leads to excessive lactic acid production.

C. Low perfusion pressure results in anaerobic metabolism, which leads to reduced lactic acid production.

D. High perfusion pressure results in anaerobic metabolism, which leads to reduced lactic acid production.

85. Appropriate tissue oxygenation depends upon adequate perfusion. Three primary factors influence perfusion. These factors are:

A. adequate heart rate, adequate fluid, and an intact vascular system.

B. adequate pump, adequate fluid, and an intact vascular system.

C. adequate pump, adequate fluid, and a dilated vascular system.

D. adequate heart rate, adequate fluid, and a dilated vascular system.

86. Which statement best describes why it is important for the EMT-Intermediate to adequately ventilate a patient with hypoperfusion or shock?

A. Increasing the oxygen concentration improves cerebral blood flow.

B. Increasing the oxygen concentration causes arterial vasoconstriction.

C. Removal of carbon dioxide is important in reducing the accumulation of body acids.

D. Removal of carbon dioxide will increase the acid and reduce the pH.

87. An increase in peripheral vascular resistance with compensated shock will be measured by a(n):

A. increase in systolic blood pressure.

B. increase in diastolic blood pressure.

C. decrease in systolic blood pressure.

D. decrease in diastolic blood pressure.

88. What effect does peripheral vasodilatation have on blood return to the heart?
    A. Blood return to the heart is decreased.
    B. Blood return to the heart is increased.
    C. Blood return to the heart is unchanged.
    D. Blood return to the heart is minimally increased.

89. Intracellular fluid accounts for what percent of total body water?
    A. 7.5%
    B. 17.5%
    C. 25%
    D. 75%

90. What is the prevalent cation in extracellular fluid?
    A. calcium
    B. magnesium
    C. sodium
    D. potassium

91. Which statement best describes the role of proteins in the body?
    A. Proteins play a major role in the production of lipids.
    B. Proteins are necessary for body growth, development, and repair.
    C. Proteins are a minor element in the building material for muscles, hair, skin, and blood.
    D. Proteins form a few hormones in the body.

92. Osmosis is best defined as movement:
    A. of water from an area of greater solute concentration to an area of lesser solute concentration.
    B. of water from an area of lesser solute concentration to an area of greater solute concentration.

    C. of solutes from an area of greater concentration to an area of lesser concentration.
    D. of solutes from an area of lesser concentration to an area of greater concentration.

93. A solution with a lower solute concentration on one side of a semi-permeable membrane when compared to a solution on the opposite side is called a:
    A. tonic solution.
    B. hypertonic solution.
    C. isotonic solution.
    D. hypotonic solution.

94. What is the chief intracellular cation?
    A. sodium
    B. calcium
    C. potassium
    D. chloride

95. The concentration of hydrogen ions in body fluid is called:
    A. carbonic acid system.
    B. acid-base balance.
    C. bicarbonate buffer system.
    D. electrolyte balance system.

96. A pH level below _____ is considered acidic.
    A. 7.50
    B. 7.45
    C. 7.40
    D. 7.35

97. Acidosis that results from hypoventilation is called:
    A. respiratory acidosis.
    B. respiratory alkalosis.
    C. metabolic acidosis.
    D. metabolic alkalosis.

98. Excessive removal of carbon dioxide by hyperventilation produces:
    A. respiratory acidosis.
    B. respiratory alkalosis.
    C. metabolic acidosis.
    D. metabolic alkalosis.

99. An accumulation of metabolic acids resulting from low perfusion states is called:
    A. respiratory acidosis.
    B. respiratory alkalosis.
    C. metabolic acidosis.
    D. metabolic alkalosis.

100. An increased intake of antacids can result in:
    A. respiratory acidosis.
    B. respiratory alkalosis.
    C. metabolic acidosis.
    D. metabolic alkalosis.

101. Hypoperfusion or shock may result in cerebral hypoxia. Which of the following is an early sign of cerebral hypoxia?
    A. a slowing pulse rate
    B. restlessness or anxiety
    C. presence of decerebrate posturing
    D. presence of decorticate posturing

102. Which of the following signs would be consistent with decompensated shock?
    A. pink color skin
    B. strong regular pulse of 90
    C. narrow pulse pressure
    D. warm, dry skin

103. Which injury would be a contraindication for the use of the PASG?
    A. a patient with a gunshot wound to the abdomen
    B. a patient with a laceration to the lower leg
    C. a patient who has been stabbed in the chest
    D. a patient with a stab wound to the abdomen

104. All of the following intravenous fluids are correctly paired with its class or form, **except**:
    A. plasma protein fraction (plasmanate)—colloid
    B. hetastarch (hespan)—colloid
    C. normal saline—crystalloid
    D. lactated Ringer's—colloid

105. Which intravenous fluid would be the initial fluid of choice in the prehospital setting for a trauma patient who requires volume replacement?
    A. lactated Ringer's
    B. 5% dextrose in water
    C. dextran
    D. hespan

106. What two parameters are monitored during fluid replacement therapy in an adult patient?
    A. pulse and pupil reaction
    B. blood pressure and pupil reaction
    C. blood pressure and body temperature
    D. pulse and blood pressure

107. You are transporting a patient from a local hospital to a regional trauma center. The patient was struck by a car an hour earlier. An intravenous solution of whole blood is being administered during your transport. The patient suddenly develops hives, palpitations, and is nauseated. You should suspect what condition?
    A. fluid overload
    B. pulmonary embolism
    C. transfusion reaction
    D. pulmonary contusion

108. What route is most commonly used for fluid replacement in the prehospital patient?
    A. oral
    B. rectal
    C. intravenous
    D. intraosseous

109. What two factors are most important in determining the speed of flow of intravenous fluids?
    A. the height of the intravenous fluid container and the size of the vein utilized.
    B. the size of the vein utilized and the length of the intravenous catheter.
    C. the length of the intravenous catheter and the height of the intravenous container.
    D. the length of the intravenous catheter and the diameter of the intravenous catheter.

110. The body is made up mostly of water, which is compartmentalized into fluids that share similar characteristics or purposes. Which one of the following has the greatest amount of water?
    A. extracellular fluid
    B. interstitial fluid
    C. intravascular fluid
    D. intracellular fluid

111. The body will move water from the interstitial spaces into the intravascular space when there is decreased circulating volume. This process can be defined as:
    A. osmosis.
    B. diffusion.
    C. active transport.
    D. mediated transport.

112. Which of the following fluids is hypertonic and will cause water to enter the intravascular compartment?
    A. 0.45% NaCl
    B. 0.9% NaCl
    C. 3% NaCl
    D. none of the above

113. Osmosis is the movement of _____ from an area of lower solute concentration to one of higher solute concentration.
    A. electrolytes
    B. water
    C. proteins
    D. red blood cells

114. Sodium moves from a higher concentration on one side of a semi-permeable membrane to a lower concentration by a process called:
    A. osmosis.
    B. diffusion.
    C. active transport.
    D. mediated transport.

115. Which of the following is pumped out of the cell by a process known as active transport?
    A. sodium
    B. potassium
    C. albumin
    D. glucose

116. Proteins play a role in which of the following?
    A. fluid tonicity
    B. immune system components
    C. antigen formation
    D. all of the above

117. Electrolytes are contained within certain spaces of the body to meet metabolic

demands. As needed they are moved from location to location by all of the following mechanism, **except**:

A. diffusion.

B. active transport.

C. forced movement.

D. mediated transport.

118. A patient presents with severe vomiting for the past 3 days. What would you expect the pH to do?

A. increase, causing metabolic acidosis

B. decrease, causing respiratory alkalosis

C. increase, causing metabolic alkalosis

D. the pH should remain the same

119. A person who is not acclimated is visiting the Colorado Rocky Mountains, and is at an elevation of 14,000 feet. Which of the following would most likely explain his acid-base condition?

A. metabolic acidosis

B. metabolic alkalosis

C. respiratory acidosis

D. respiratory alkalosis

120. How do proteins influence the concentrations of water across a semi-permeable membrane?

A. They force water to leave spaces containing proteins.

B. They are large molecules which help keep water within that space.

C. They are small molecules which rapidly leave spaces, taking water with them.

D. They are only located outside the vascular spaces, drawing water towards them.

121. A patient has overdosed on a narcotic medication. His vitals are: B/P 100/58, HR 86, and RR 8 and shallow. His primary acid-base disturbance is:

A. metabolic acidosis.

B. metabolic alkalosis.

C. respiratory acidosis.

D. respiratory alkalosis.

122. A drop in the level of hydrogen ions in the body will result in a(n) _____ in the level of carbonic acid, and in turn, carbon dioxide levels will _____.

A. increase, decrease

B. decrease, increase

C. increase, increase

D. decrease, decrease

123. Compensated metabolic acidosis will cause the respiratory rate to:

A. decrease.

B. increase.

C. initially increase and then slow down.

D. not change whatsoever.

124. Which of the following would best describe the body's response to metabolic alkalosis?

A. There will be an increase in the respiratory rate.

B. There will be a decrease in the respiratory rate.

C. There will be an increase in hydrogen ion excretion by the kidneys.

D. There will be an increase in bicarbonate ion retention by the kidneys.

125. One principle problem for a patient in shock is the excessive production of acid. This production of acid is primarily a result of:

A. decreased production of pyruvate.

B. increased activity of the sodium/potassium pump.

C. the liberation of lysosomes.

D. a shift to anaerobic metabolism.

126. A patient has sustained a laceration to the forearm from a bar fight. Upon arrival, the patient is still bleeding profusely. You quickly control the bleed, and during your assessment you find the following vitals: HR 110, RR 30, B/P 110/88. Skin is cool, diaphoretic, and pale to the extremities. Your patient is in what stage of shock?
    A. irreversible shock
    B. progressive shock
    C. compensated shock
    D. decompensated shock

127. When a person is suffering from distributive shock, the blood pressure characteristically drops because of:
    A. an increase in the heart rate.
    B. a drop in the cardiac preload.
    C. severe vasoconstriction.
    D. an increase in stroke volume.

128. Anaerobic metabolism may be reduced by:
    A. decreasing cardiac preload.
    B. decreasing afterload.
    C. widening the pulse pressure.
    D. improving the FiO_2.

129. Your patient has lost an estimated 1,000 ml of blood from a penetrating thoracic injury. What should guide the volume of fluid administered to the patient?
    A. the diastolic blood pressure
    B. the pulse pressure and heart rate
    C. radial pulse and systolic blood pressure
    D. carotid pulse and diastolic blood pressure

130. You are providing aggressive fluid resuscitation to a patient who has lost a large amount of blood due to multiple gunshot wounds. The volume to be infused is:
    A. 20 ml/kg, and then reassess.
    B. 2,000 ml, and then reassess.
    C. 40 ml/kg, and then reassess.
    D. 4,000 ml, and then reassess.

131. In which patient would the PASG be contraindicated?
    A. burn shock
    B. hypovolemic shock
    C. cardiogenic shock
    D. septic shock

132. Which of the following injuries may most likely lead to hypoxia and hypercapnia?
    A. fractured pelvis
    B. abdominal bleeding
    C. fractured femur
    D. flail segment

133. The most reliable indicator of cerebral perfusion status in shock is:
    A. the level of consciousness.
    B. a Glasgow Coma Score over 8.
    C. a normal pupillary response.
    D. moist mucosal membranes.

134. Why is 5% dextrose in water not a preferred solution for volume expansion in a hypovolemic patient?
    A. because the glucose raises metabolic rate
    B. because it draws fluid into the vascular space
    C. because it rapidly leaves the vascular space
    D. none of the above

135. A patient has rapidly received about 1,500 ml of solution for hypovolemic shock. Upon reassessment you discover inspiratory crackles in the lung bases. You should:
    A. repeat the fluid bolus.
    B. shut off the IV.
    C. initiate another IV.
    D. turn the IV rate down to KVO.

136. Which of the following would allow the fastest administration of solution in a hypovolemic trauma patient?
    A. a 14-gauge angio with a microdrip administration set
    B. a 22-gauge angio with a microdrip administration set
    C. a 16-gauge angio with a macrodrip administration set
    D. a 18-gauge angio with a macrodrip administration set

137. When infusing fluids in a trauma patient, there is stretch of the myocardial fibers from the increased preload. As this stretch occurs, the force of contraction _____.
    A. increases
    B. rapidly decreases
    C. progressively decreases
    D. does not change

138. How does the pneumatic anti-shock garment (PASG) increase systolic blood pressure?
    A. by decreasing afterload
    B. by increasing systemic vascular resistance.
    C. by decreasing preload
    D. by decreasing afterload

139. The baroreceptors monitor:
    A. carbon dioxide levels.
    B. oxygen levels.
    C. blood pressure.
    D. the heart rate.

140. Arterial blood passing through capillary beds will:
    A. release oxygen and carbon dioxide.
    B. pick up oxygen and release carbon dioxide.
    C. pick up carbon dioxide and excess oxygen.
    D. release oxygen and pick up carbon dioxide.

141. If you want to administer fluid to a patient without increasing intravascular volume, you would infuse:
    A. a hypertonic solution.
    B. a hypotonic solution.
    C. an isotonic solution.
    D. none of the above

142. A fluid like lactated Ringer's is used in the prehospital environment for:
    A. head injury patients.
    B. hypothermic patients.
    C. cardiac patients.
    D. dehydrated patients.

143. A significant increase in hydrostatic pressure in the pulmonary capillary network will have which of the following effects on oxygenation?
    A. It will improve oxygenation of tissue due to an increase in perfusion pressures.
    B. Hypoxia will occur from leakage of fluid into the alveolar-capillary interface which will interfere with gas diffusion.
    C. It will reduce the amount of gas flowing into the alveoli from the terminal bronchiole.
    D. Oxygen diffusion is improved because of the increased number of red blood cells in the alveolar capillary interface.

144. Oxygen and carbon dioxide will diffuse:
    A. from areas of high concentration to low concentration.
    B. more easily across the alveolar capillary membrane with an increase in interstitial fluid in the space.
    C. from the capillary bed into the alveoli.
    D. only in the presence of an acidic environment in the cell.

145. You arrive on scene and find a patient with a suspected intra-abdominal bleed from blunt trauma. The blood pressure is 102/84 mmHg. The skin is pale, cool, and clammy. The diastolic blood pressure reflects:
    A. decompensatory shock.
    B. an increase in cardiac output.
    C. an increase in systemic vascular resistance.
    D. a widening in the pulse pressure.

146. Which of the following is an early sign of an increase in systemic vascular resistance?
    A. an increase in heart rate
    B. a decreased mental status
    C. pale, cool, clammy skin
    D. a decrease in systolic blood pressure

147. A decrease in venous volume will:
    A. increase stroke volume.
    B. trigger peripheral vasodilation.
    C. increase cerebral perfusion pressure.
    D. reduce preload in the left ventricle.

148. Which of the following is a cation?
    A. chloride
    B. calcium
    C. bicarbonate
    D. phosphate

149. Bicarbonate is:
    A. a major anion.
    B. an acidodic solution.
    C. the primary carrier of oxygen in blood.
    D. a cation found in the body.

150. Which of the following would move fastest across a semi-permeable membrane?
    A. albumin
    B. electrolytes

C. water
D. dextrose

151. If a hypotonic fluid was infused, the fluid would have which of the following effects?
    A. It would draw fluid into the vessel.
    B. It would leave the vascular space quickly.
    C. It would not move but stay in the vascular space.
    D. It would dehydrate the interstitial space.

152. What type of fluid would cause the quickest increase in intravascular volume when infused?
    A. hypotonic
    B. isotonic
    C. hypertonic
    D. normotonic

153. Eventually the normal saline or lactated Ringer's that was infused in a trauma patient will move out of the vascular space. This is primarily because of:
    A. diffusion of the charged particles.
    B. osmosis of the plasma proteins.
    C. active transport of dextrose molecules.
    D. non-permeable capillary membranes.

154. The sodium/potassium pump is an example of:
    A. facilitated diffusion.
    B. osmosis.
    C. diffusion.
    D. active transport.

155. Which of following statements about active transport is false.
    A. It can move molecules from an area of low concentration to high concentration.
    B. It does not require energy to move molecules.

C. It is typically faster than diffusion.

D. It can move larger molecules across membranes.

156. Which of the following occurs as the carbon dioxide level increases in the blood?

A. The pH value increases indicating alkalosis.

B. The PaO_2 level will increase from hypoventilation.

C. The carbonic acid increase will decrease the pH value.

D. The pH value will increase due to a decrease in hydrogen ions.

157. A patient who has a respiratory rate of 6/minute most likely would be in:

A. metabolic alkalosis.

B. ketoacidosis.

C. respiratory acidosis.

D. respiratory alkalosis.

158. The physician in the emergency department tells you that the patient you brought in earlier had a pH of 7.34, a PaO_2 of 98 mmHg, and a $PaCO_2$ of 38 mmHg. You would interpret these blood gases and conclude that the patient is in:

A. respiratory acidosis and metabolic alkalosis.

B. respiratory alkalosis and metabolic acidosis.

C. respiratory acidosis only.

D. metabolic acidosis only.

159. You are treating a patient with a self-inflicted gunshot wound to the abdomen. His skin is pale, cool, and clammy. Vitals are: BP 78/58, RR 22/minute, and HR 128/minute. He is most likely in:

A. respiratory acidosis.

B. metabolic acidosis.

C. respiratory alkalosis.

D. metabolic alkalosis.

160. You are managing a 2-year-old child who has ingested approximately 30 aspirin. The mother thought he was in his room taking a nap when she discovered him after about two hours. Based on the substance ingested, you would expect the respiratory rate and depth to be:

A. increased.

B. decreased.

C. labored.

D. not affected.

161. You arrive on scene to find a patient who has been ill with the flu for the last few days. She states she has been vomiting profusely since becoming sick. She complains of severe weakness and muscle aches. What would you estimate her pH to be?

A. greater than 7.40

B. 7.40

C. 7.35

D. less than 7.35

162. The immediate response of the body to a decrease in blood pressure is innervated through which of the following?

A. hormonal response from the sympathetic nervous system

B. vagal nerve impulses

C. direct neural stimulation from the sympathetic nervous system

D. parasympathetic nervous stimulation and release of acetylcholine

163. The cascade effect of nervous system innervation and the hormonal response seen in the compensatory phase of shock is primarily initiated by:
    A. an increase in systemic vascular resistance.
    B. a decrease in the PaO_2 recognized by the medullary chemoreceptor.
    C. a change in the perfusion pressure in the kidney.
    D. a decrease in the volume of blood and pressure found in the aortic arch and carotid bodies.

164. An increase in the stretch of the baroreceptor would cause which of the following effects?
    A. an increase in the heart rate and stroke volume
    B. a decrease in peripheral vascular resistance
    C. vasoconstricion of the systemic vessels
    D. an increase in stroke volume and peripheral resistance

165. The best clinical indicator of early peripheral vasoconstriction is measured by assessing the:
    A. heart rate.
    B. skin color, temperature, and condition.
    C. systolic blood pressure.
    D. pupillary response to light.

166. Which of the following would best represent a blood pressure of a patient in compensatory shock?
    A. 70/50 mmHg
    B. 102/52 mmHg
    C. 108/84 mmHg
    D. 158/60 mmHg

167. Which of the following would be an indication to apply and inflate the pneumatic anti-shock garment?
    A. a patient who has suffered multiple thoracic and abdominal stab wounds and has a blood pressure of 100/76 mmHg
    B. a patient with a suspected head injury whose pressure is 50/30 mmHg
    C. a patient with instability to the pelvis, abdominal tenderness and rigidity, and a left femur fracture whose blood pressure is 74/52 mmHg
    D. a patient with a gunshot wound to the epigastric region, a large laceration to the left lower leg, hemoptysis, and rectal bleeding who has a blood pressure of 68/48 mmHg

168. Which of the following fluids would exert a hypertonic effect?
    A. lactated Ringer's
    B. normal saline
    C. packed cells
    D. human serum albumin

169. When infusing crystalloid solutions in an elderly patient, it is important to constantly monitor for fluid overload by frequently checking blood pressure and:
    A. assessing the breath sounds in the lower lobes of the lungs.
    B. checking for pitting edema in the lower extremities.
    C. watching for bradycardia.
    D. assessing for an increase in the pulse oximetry reading.

170. In the hypovolemic patient who has a suspected intra-abdominal hemorrhage you should run the fluid wide open until:

A. at least 20 ml/kg of fluid is delivered.

B. you get a systolic blood pressure of at least 90 mmHg.

C. the heart rate decreases by 10 beats/minute.

D. there is no orthostatic drop in blood pressure.

171. You arrive on scene and find a patient who has sliced his forearm on a piece of glass while replacing a window. He is bleeding profusely upon your arrival. You control the bleeding with direct pressure. His vital signs are BP 88/68 mmHg, HR 118, RR 22 with good tidal volume. His skin is pale, cool, and clammy. Your treatment should consist of:

A. administering O_2 by non-rebreather and initiating an IV of normal saline running at 20 ml/kg until the systolic blood pressure returns to greater than 100 mmHg.

B. applying a nasal cannula at 6 lpm, initiating an IV of lactated Ringer's, and infusing wide open until the systolic BP reaches 90 mmHg then cut it back to TKO.

C. inserting an oropharyngeal airway, beginning bag-valve-mask ventilation, and initiating an IV of normal saline en route run at a TKO rate.

D. applying a non-rebreather and initiating an IV of lactated Ringer's running wide open until the radial pulse returns then cut it back to TKO.

172. You are instructed by medical direction to infuse 1,000 ml of normal saline in a trauma patient as quickly as possible. You would select which of the following equipment?

A. an 18-gauge catheter with a 10-drop macrodrip set

B. a 16-gauge catheter with a 20-drop macrodrip set

C. a 20-gauge catheter with a blood solution set

D. a 14-gauge catheter with a 10-drop macrodrip set

173. You have started an IV line of normal saline in a trauma patient and have it running at a wide open rate. The patient experiences a sudden onset of fever, chills, headache, nausea and begins to vomit. You should

A. suspect the shock is worsening and infuse the fluid faster.

B. immediately stop the infusion and discontinue it and restart a new IV in the opposite extremity using new tubing, solution, and catheter suspecting a pyrogenic reaction.

C. apply pressure to the IV site and remove the catheter because of extravasation of the fluid into the interstitial spaces.

D. apply warm compresses to the IV site and request antibiotic therapy upon your arrival at the hospital for thrombophlebitis.

174. Which of the following pH values would reflect a decrease in hydrogen ion concentration in the blood?

A. 7.48

B. 7.40

C. 7.38

D. 7.20

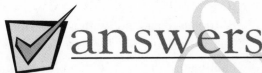

answers & rationales

1.

B. Proteins have numerous responsibilities in the body. One of them is to maintain colloidal osmotic pressure, while influencing the amount of water crossing a semipermeable membrane. Since proteins are larger molecules that do not cross membranes easily, they help maintain normal fluid distribution in the body. *(1.8.12)*

2.

C. A burn patient would benefit from a hypertonic solution because the hypertonicity of the IV fluids would draw water from the interstitial spaces back into the vasculature. Remember also that a burn patient loses a large amount of fluids to the tissues as a result of the burn. A hypertonic solution can also help reduce the swelling seen in severe burn patients. *(1.8.14)*

3.

A. Albumin is a large protein that usually needs transportation across the membrane. Active transport is when the body expends energy in order to move a molecule or electrolyte across a semipermeable membrane. This is done either because it goes against its concentration gradient, or because the molecule is large. Glucose needs assistance as well from insulin, but it does not require energy, this is known as facilitated transport. *(1.8.16)*

4.

B. The blood buffer system is the initial mechanism the body uses to buffer an increase in hydrogen ion concentration. In this situation, the hydrogen is combined with bicarbonate ions to form carbonic acid (a weaker acid). Excretion of hydrogen from the kidneys can occur, but it is a very slow process. *(1.8.19)*

5.

C. Respiratory acidosis occurs when the $PaCO_2$ levels become elevated beyond 45 mmHg in the arterial circulation. This occurs as a result of diminished alveolar ventilation because CO_2 is eliminated during exhalation. With any decrease in minute ventilation, a drop in respiratory rate and depth, CO_2 levels rise. *(1.8.20a)*

6.

B. Baroreceptors are special pressure receptors found only in the aortic arch and carotid bodies. These sensors monitor the degree of arterial pressure and provide feedback to the vasomotor center in the medulla regarding the degree of arterial tone. Chemoreceptors monitor O_2, CO_2, and hydrogen levels for respiratory efficiency. *(1.8.22)*

7.

A. A decrease in preload decreases coronary artery perfusion, which occurs only during diastole. *(1.8.25)*

8.

A. As long as there is a radial pulse, perfusion pressures are considered to generally be at a resuscitation level that is acceptable. If however, the patient continues to loose blood to the point where compensatory mechanisms fail, the radial pulse will disappear. If this happens, it generally correlates with the patient progressing from compensatory shock to decompensatory shock. *(1.8.26)*

9.

B. Concentrations of gases in the body travel down what is known as it's "partial pressure gradient." This is the difference from one side to the other, or in other words, oxygen will go from an area of high concentration to low concentration. Active transport, mediated transport, and osmosis refers to the movement of molecules or water, respectively. *(1.8.3)*

10.

A. A negative feedback system for shock patients is closure of precapillary sphincters. This will direct blood away from the non-essential vascular beds of the periphery back to core perfusion. This effectively decreases the size of the vascular "container" which brings the amount of volume and the "container" size closer to normal proportions. The body tries, as long as possible, to maintain perfusion to the heart, lungs, brain, and kidneys. *(1.8.8)*

11.

D. Because of a diminishment in preload (presumably caused by pulmonary vessel damage from the assault), there will be less blood for the heart to pump out. This will result in a drop in stroke volume that will subsequently cause a drop in cardiac output and blood pressure. *(1.8.9)*

12.

A. Administering a fluid bolus to a hypovolemic patient will provide more volume in the venous system, which will result in an increased preload. Heart rate and contractility may be moderately enhanced with the increased preload, but that is not the major benefit of IV therapy. Afterload refers to the degree of arterial tone the heart needs to contract against. *(1.8.6)*

13.

C. The treatment is to slow the IV rate down to KVO and consult medical control. Volume expansion is necessary for a hypovolemic patient in shock. Be careful however, not to overhydrate them. If that occurs you will note inspiratory crackles and JVD. *(1.8.29)*

14.

A. When providing fluid resuscitation, use the most appropriate equipment that will allow a rapid infusion of volume. This should include a large bore angiocatheter, an isotonic solution, and macrodrip administration, or even a blood solution set. *(1.8.34)*

15.

B. Damage to the mitral valve will allow regurgitation of blood backwards through the left atrium, pulmonary veins, and into the perialveolar capillary beds. Here, hydrostatic pressure will increase to a point where fluid is forced into the alveoli causing pulmonary edema. *(1.8.8)*

16.

C. An increase in the force of ventricular contraction will cause improvement in the stroke volume, this leads to better cardiac output and an increased systolic blood pressure. *(1.8.6)*

17.

D. Dyspnea associated with inspiratory crackles is very characteristic of pump failure. One role of the EMT-I is to delineate the different presentations of shock, either a volume, pump, or container problem. There may be associated hypotension which is not treated with fluid bolus. *(1.8.28)*

18.

A. Any patient who cannot control their own airway should have it done artificially by endotracheal intubation in the absence of a gag reflex. Immobilization should always occur based on mechanism of injury, and medical control may still authorize the use of the AED. Volume expansion should occur with an isotonic volume expander such as normal saline or lactated Ringer's. *(1.8.35)*

19.

A. High flow oxygen would be the most beneficial option for this patient. This individual appears to have a lacerated spleen and is becoming hypovolemic. Human cellular function is dependent upon adequate oxygenation via the red blood cells (hemoglobin). Because the hemorrhage is internal, hemorrhage control is difficult. Subsequently, the EMT-Intermediate must saturate the remaining red blood cells with oxygen in an attempt to maximize delivery of oxygen to the body tissues. Fluid replacement is important, but will not deliver increased amounts of oxygen to the individual cells. *(1.8.4)*

20.

B. Systemic vascular resistance relates to the degree of pressure that exists in the peripheral vasculature when not influenced by cardiac output. Therefore, an appropriate measure of this pressure can be estimated by using the diastolic number obtained in the blood pressure. Consequently, the systolic pressure is incorrect in that this is a measurement of pressure created by actual cardiac output. Also, the palpation of a radial pulse is a function of cardiac output and is incorrect. The pulse pressure is an indicator of the degree to which a body is compensating during illness or injury. *(1.8.8)*

21.

A. Sodium is the chief extracellular ion and is the principle electrolyte in regulating water balance. Electrolytes are not used for fuel by the body but rather work with other nutrients to aid in body function. Sodium does not play a direct role in cellular metabolization. *(1.8.11)*

22.

D. Through osmosis, water will move from the extracellular space into the cellular compartment. This occurs so as to equalize the concentrations of the solution on both sides of the cellular membrane. Because of the difference in concentration, water will not be displaced from the intracellular compartment. Potassium cannot actively cross the cellular membrane, so the potassium will remain unchanged. *(1.8.13)*

23.

A. Diffusion is the mechanism responsible for the movement of oxygen molecules from the arterial blood into the intracellular space. Since this movement does not require any supplemental energy, it cannot be described as active transport. Osmosis pertains to the movement of a solvent such as water between areas of higher and lower concentrations. Saturation pertains to a solvents ability to effectively dissolve and carry a certain amount of a solute. *(1.8.15)*

24.

B. Renal function absorbs or excretes sodium ions to maintain the body's concentration of the electrolyte. Pulmonary function is not applicable here in that this system regulates oxygen and carbon dioxide levels. The liver detoxifies substances, and the vasomotor center regulates blood pressure *(1.8.17)*

25.

D. Carbon dioxide influences the relative acidity of the blood. The typical range for $PaCO_2$ is 35 to 45 mmHg. A $PaCO_2$ of 31 mmHg represents a low concentration of carbon dioxide and indicates the blood is in an alkalotic state. This is reflected as an increase in the blood pH. A decrease in the pH would indicate an acidiotic state caused by an increase in CO2. A decrease in saturated hemoglobin would not directly affect the blood pH. *(1.8.20)*

26.

D. Extensive vomiting results in a loss of hydrogen cations from the body. Such a loss causes an increase in pH and results in metabolic alkalosis. Respiratory alkalosis is a result of a disproportionate loss of CO_2 through the respiratory system. Metabolic acidosis would indicate the loss of a base or an unbuffered increase in the hydrogen cation. Hypervolemia is incorrect in that this suggests an overloading of fluid. *(1.8.20)*

27.

C. Neural stimuli initiated by the baroreceptors causes pronounced smooth muscle contraction or relaxation of the arterioles, resulting in changes in the blood pressure. The vena cava, venules, and capillaries contain little to no smooth muscle so minimal or no contraction/relaxation occurs. *(1.8.23)*

28.

A. Prior to transport, first you must begin bag-valve-mask ventilation with supplemental oxygen connected to the reservoir. Secondly, the patient must be fully immobilized to a backboard. The fractures will be somewhat splinted by the backboard and are not a major concern. *(1.8.31)*

29.

C. The continued needs of this patient include rapid transport and the continued administration of lactated Ringer's. The administration of lactated Ringer's with its associated positive effects are only temporary in that only volume expansion has been achieved. Volume expansion does not replace the loss of the red blood cells which serve to transport oxygen to the individual cells. Once a radial pulse is regained, reduce the fluid administration so not to promote further bleeding. *(1.8.32)*

30.

B. Regaining the radial pulse would indicate that the peripheral perfusion is improving. The presence of diaphoresis would suggest continued cellular hypoxia through the innervation of the sympathetic nervous system. Warm skin is not the best indication because this may suggest body heated volume expansion. This is not a guarantee of alleviated anaerobic metabolism. In addition, the sympathetic nervous system can maintain the blood pressure via vasoconstriction in a compensatory effort. *(1.8.33)*

31.

A. The greatest limitation to the rate at which a volume can be administered is the catheter lumen. The greater the diameter, the greater the volume of fluid that can pass through the cannula on a second by second basis. As the veins are typically elastic in nature, the size of the vein will not limit the rate of infusion. The type of crystalloid infused and the size of the bag will not influence the rate at which the fluid passes through the IV cannula. *(1.8.34)*

32.

B. The initial step in glucose metabolism by the cell (glycolysis) is an anaerobic process which results in the formation of pyruvic acid. If oxygen is not available to continue the process, pyruvic acid will convert to lactic acid. *(1.8.1)*

33.

D. Administering oxygen and ventilatory support are critical to the management of shock. Hypoxia triggers the release of vasodilators as a compensatory mechanism in shock. This increases localized blood flow but decreases systemic vascular resistance resulting in low blood pressures. Acidosis causes depression of the central nervous system including the vasomotor center. *(1.8.5)*

34.

A. Cardiac output is decreased when hypovolemia reduces preload, the blood available to the pump. Adequate tissue perfusion is dependent on a functional and well-oxygenated pump (heart), adequate volume (blood), and an intact container (blood vessels). The fluid-container-volume ratio must match. *(1.8.9)*

35.

B. Plasma is an extracellular fluid, which comprises one third of body fluid. Interstitial fluid, found in the microscopic spaces between tissue cells, includes aqueous humor, cerebrospinal fluid, and lymph. *(1.8.10)*

36.

A. Hemoglobin plays a critical role by transporting oxygen in the blood. Other important physiologic functions of proteins include immunological (interleukin, antibodies), structural (collagen), and catalytic (lipase). *(1.8.12)*

37.

C. Administering a hypotonic solution will cause water to move into the red blood cells causing them to swell and eventually burst. *(1.8.14)*

38.

A. The sodium-potassium pump in myocardial cells is an example of active transport. Active transport is a biochemical process where a substance is moved across a cell membrane, often against an osmotic gradient, using energy. *(1.8.16)*

39.

B. The dynamic relationship is known as acid-base balance. The production of hydrogen ions (acids) through metabolism and other chemical processes must be balanced by the buffer system, the exhalation of carbon dioxide, and kidney excretion to ensure homeostasis and survival. *(1.8.18)*

40.

D. Metabolic acidosis can result from the excess production of lactic acid, diabetes, or diarrhea. In metabolic acidosis, the pH level is decreased while the $PaCO_2$ level remains normal. Management of metabolic acidosis consists primarily of ventilation to increase the elimination of carbon dioxide. *(1.8.20)*

41.

C. Compensatory mechanisms for shock are mediated by the sympathetic nervous system and the release of various substances after the decrease in blood volume is recognized by baroreceptors. These mechanisms include vasoconstriction of the arterioles and venules of the skin, initiation of the renin-angiotension pathway to increase blood pressure, and increased reabsorption of sodium and water to restore blood volume. *(1.8.24)*

42.

A. While the administration of any solution will cause an initial increase in circulatory volume, 5% dextrose in water is a poor choice for fluid replacement because the glucose is quickly metabolized resulting in an increase in free water. This free water is hypotonic and it will dilute the remaining blood volume and leave the intravascular space quickly. *(1.8.32)*

43.

B. Although protocols may set parameters for fluid replacement, the flow rate for fluid replacement should be based on the patient's response to treatment as evidenced by improving vital signs, mental status, and return of peripheral pulses. Once stabilized, you should continue to closely monitor your patient's status being alert to the presence of signs and symptoms of developing pulmonary edema. *(1.8.33)*

44.

C. Although the predictable location of central veins permits rapid access in the field setting, peripheral vasculature is generally preferred. The cannulation of central lines often takes longer than peripheral access. It also requires the use of a sterile procedure, has a higher complication rate, and usually requires x-ray confirmation of placement. *(1.8.34)*

45.

B. In poor perfusion states and hypoxia, an inadequate amount of oxygen is available to the cells, resulting in anaerobic metabolism. You can increase perfusion by positioning the patient, replacing the lost volume, and hemorrhage control. Hypoxia can be decreased by administering oxygen, intubation, and ventilation. *(1.8.2)*

46.

A. Diffusion does not require energy and is the movement of gas from an area of higher partial pressure concentration to an area of lower partial pressure concentration. Osmosis is the movement of water across a semi-permeable membrane from a lesser concentration to an area of greater concentration. Active transport is the movement of a substance across a cell membrane against the osmotic gradient and requires energy. Facilitated transport requires the assistance of a helper protein on the surface of the cell membrane. This type of transport may or may not require energy. *(1.8.3)*

47.

A. An increase in either stroke volume or heart rate will improve the patient's cardiac output. Decreasing the stroke volume or the heart rate will cause a decrease in cardiac output. Decreased preload and an increase in systemic vascular resistance will decrease cardiac output. *(1.8.6)*

48.

B. Cardiac preload is increased when the venous side of the vascular system contracts, decreasing capacitance (the size of the container). *(1.8.7)*

49.

D. The intracellular fluid makes up 75 percent of the body's total water content. Intravascular fluid makes up 7.5 percent of the total body water. Interstitial fluid makes up 17.5 percent of the total body water. Both the intravascular and the interstitial fluid combined make up a total of 25 percent of the total body water that is contained in the extracellular space. *(1.8.10)*

50.

A. Potassium is the most prevalent cation in the intracellular fluid. Calcium plays a major role in muscle contraction. Sodium is the most prevalent cation in the extracellular fluid and plays a major role in water distribution. Magnesium is necessary for many biochemical processes. *(1.8.11)*

51.

D. Proteins, specifically helper proteins, assist certain molecules to cross the cell membrane by binding with the molecule, and then changes its configuration to enter the cell where it releases the molecule. Glucose is an example of a molecule that enters the cell by facilitated diffusion. *(1.8.12)*

52.

A. Diffusion does not require energy to move the solute across the cell membrane from a higher concentration to a lower concentration. Osmosis is the movement of water across a semi-permeable membrane so as to dilute an area of higher solute (electrolyte). Active transport is the movement of a substance across a cell membrane against the osmotic gradient. Facilitated diffusion requires the assistance of helper proteins to transport molecules into the cells. *(1.8.15)*

53.

D. Active transport is the movement of a substance across a cell membrane against the osmotic gradient. Centrifugation is the mechanism of separating plasma from formed elements. Facilitated transport requires the use of helper proteins to transport substances across the cell membrane. *(1.8.16)*

54.

A. Sodium is the most prevalent cation in the extracellular fluid and it plays a major role in the distribution of water. Potassium is the most prevalent cation in the intracellular fluid. Phosphate is an anion not a cation and it acts as a buffer primarily in the intracellular space. Chloride is not a cation, it is an anion and it plays a major role in fluid balance. *(1.8.17)*

55.

D. A pH of 7.27 is considered acidotic. The normal accepted pH range for an adult is 7.35 to 7.45. Below 7.35 is considered acidotic and above 7.45 is considered alkalotic. *(1.8.18)*

56.

B. The respiratory system will intervene to change the hydrogen ion concentration if the bicarbonate buffer system has not changed the pH significantly. The respiratory system lowers the pH by eliminating carbon dioxide through an increase in breathing rate. The renal system can regulate the body pH for hours or days in order to bring the pH back to normal. *(1.8.19)*

57.

D. These signs are indicative of a patient that is suffering from respiratory acidosis which is caused by retention of CO_2 from poor ventilation. Metabolic alkalosis would have decreased H^+, H_2CO_3, and normal CO_2, and usually caused by the administration of diuretics or prolonged vomiting. Metabolic acidosis can result from excessive diarrhea and diabetes, and results in an increase in H^+, H_2CO_3, and normal CO_2. Respiratory alkalosis results from excessive elimination of CO_2. *(1.8.20a)*

58.

C. Respiratory alkalosis is the result of excessive elimination of CO_2. This can be caused by hyperventilation related to anxiety. Metabolic alkalosis occurs less frequently than metabolic acidosis and can be caused by prolonged vomiting or overdosing a patient on sodium bicarbonate. Metabolic acidosis results from the production of metabolic acids such as lactic acid which can be caused by anaerobic metabolism. Respiratory acidosis is caused by retention of CO_2 resulting from poor ventilation. *(1.8.20b)*

59.

A. Metabolic acidosis can be caused by prolonged hypoperfusion or hypoxia at the cellular level. It can also be caused by diabetic ketoacidosis, poisonings, and serious infection. Hypoventilation and the retention of carbon dioxide increasing hydrogen ions will cause respiratory acidosis. Too much bicarbonate ions from ingestion of excessive amounts of antacids will cause metabolic alkalosis. Hyperventilation that eliminates CO_2 resulting in the loss of hydrogen ions will cause respiratory alkalosis. *(1.8.20c)*

60.

D. Metabolic alkalosis can be caused by vomiting and/or administration of drugs. Treatment usually consists of treating the cause such as vomiting. In respiratory acidosis, the pH is decreased and the CO_2 level is increased. In respiratory alkalosis, the pH is increased and the CO_2 level is decreased. In metabolic acidosis, the pH is decreased and the CO_2 is normal. *(1.8.20d)*

61.

A. All of these are associated with decompensated shock, as well as blood supply to essential organs diminishes and blood pressure falls. *(1.8.25)*

62.

C. When assessing the patient's perfusion status, if a carotid pulse is felt, the systolic blood pressure is estimated at 60 mmHg. If the femoral pulse is felt, the systolic blood pressure is estimated at 70 mmHg. When the radial pulse is felt, the systolic blood pressure is estimated at 80 mmHg. These are controversial estimates and may help you approximate the blood pressure. *(1.8.26)*

63.

D. This patient is in decompensated shock and needs to be rapidly and aggressively managed. This patient needs to be ventilated immediately. Also, this patient will need fluid replacement using a 14-gauge catheter. *(1.8.29)*

64.

C. The two absolute contraindications to the use of the PASG are pulmonary edema and penetrating neck or chest trauma. Active bleeding may be controlled with the direct pressure applied by the PASG. Fractures to the lower extremities can be splinted with the PASG while still gaining the other benefits. *(1.8.30)*

65.

D. Dextran 40 is a colloid solution with large sugar molecules and osmotic properties. Dextran will remain in the intravascular space for an extended period of time. Colloids attract water into the intravascular space by increasing the colloid osmotic pressure which helps expand the volume. D5W is a hypotonic glucose solution that does not expand the fluid in the intravascular space. *(1.8.32a)*

66.

C. Lactated Ringer's is not compatible with whole blood. Since it is likely that whole blood will be administered at the hospital, it is recommended that two IV lines be started. At least one IV should be normal saline where whole blood can be given, if necessary. *(1.8.32b)*

67.

D. These are all signs of circulation overload and can cause great harm or even death to your patient. As soon as you notice these symptoms immediately adjust the flow rate to a KVO. Thrombophlebitis is inflammation of the vein and is more common when the IV therapy is long term. Air embolism is when air is allowed to enter to vein. *(1.8.33a)*

68.

A. By lowering the bag, gravity will allow the blood to flow from the vein into the tubing, thus confirming that the IV is patent. Compressing the bag will not insure that the IV is in the lumen of the vein and may cause further damage if the IV has infiltrated. Replacing the constricting band on the arm will not permit you to check for patentcy, furthermore, this will reduce venous flow and cause the flow to cease. If the bag is above the IV site and the flow ceases, the IV is not patent. *(1.8.33b)*

69.

C. The greatest amount of volume can be delivered through the 14-gauge, 5-cm catheter. A lower gauge number represents a larger diameter catheter which will deliver larger amounts of fluid. A shorter catheter will deliver more fluid than a longer catheter. *(1.8.34a)*

70.

D. The external jugular or antecubital fossa are both large veins and are considered peripheral. The external jugular will accept a large catheter like a 14 gauge. Internal jugular vein cannulation is not a prehospital skill. *(1.8.34b)*

71.

A. Calcium, magnesium, potassium, and sodium are the major cations of the body. The most frequent occurring anions are bicarbonate, chloride, and phosphate. *(1.8.11)*

72.

B. Osmosis is the movement of a solvent (water) across a semi-permeable membrane from an area of lower solute concentration to an area of higher solute concentration until both sides are in equilibrium. *(1.8.13)*

73.

A. Diffusion is the movement of solutes (molecules) across the semi-permeable membrane from an area of higher concentration to an area of lower concentration, until both sides are equal. Diffusion involves particles, like electrolytes, whereas osmosis involves water. *(1.8.15)*

74.

D. Sodium is the chief extracellular ion. Potassium is the chief intracellular ion. *(1.8.17)*

75.

D. The respiratory system regulates the amount of carbon dioxide in the body. The bicarbonate system acts to regulate the amount of hydrogen ions available. The kidneys excrete either bicarbonate ions or hydrogen ions. *(1.8.19)*

76.

B. Metabolic alkalosis is the excessive loss of hydrogen ions from the body. Secondary to the loss of hydrogen ions, there may be an increase of other elemental ions, because of several different causes like administration of diuretics and excessive ingestion of alkaline drugs. *(1.8.20d)*

77.

B. Inadequate cellular oxygenation produces metabolism that is anaerobic. When oxygen is not available, tissues cannot be perfused properly, acids accumulate and cellular death will occur. *(1.8.2)*

78.

D. An increase in stroke volume or heart rate or both can increase cardiac output. In the early (compensated) stage of shock, increased cardiac output can be detected by an increasing pulse rate. *(1.8.6)*

79.

D. If the blood pressure falls, the baroreceptors stimulate the sympathetic nervous system. The heart rate and cardiac contractility are both increased along with an increase in systemic vascular resistance. *(1.8.21)*

80.

D. In decompensated shock the blood supply, and consequently the oxygen supply, to the organs decreases and the blood pressure begins to fall. The pulse and respirations continue to increase. The patient's level of consciousness deteriorates to confusion, and eventually coma. *(1.8.25)*

81.

D. Whole blood is the most desirable fluid replacement. It contains hemaglobin and other essential proteins. However, it is not a practical choice in the prehospital setting. While Plasmanate would be the next choice, colloids are not typically used in the prehospital setting, either due to their expense and short shelf-life. The solution of choice in the prehospital setting is an isotonic crystalloid. *(1.8.32)*

82.

C.
$$\frac{1\ ml}{60\ gtts} \times \frac{45\ gtts}{minutes} \times 90\ mins = 67.5\ ml \quad \textit{(1.8.33)}$$

83.

A. The antecubital fossa and external jugular veins are the ideal site for fluid volume replacement. The larger diameter of both of these veins compared to the veins of the hand and distal portion of the arm make these veins more suitable for resuscitation. *(1.8.34)*

84.

A. Low perfusion states (hypoperfusion) or shock leads to a reduction in oxygen transported to body cells. Normal metabolic processes utilize oxygen to degrade pyruvic acid into carbon dioxide, water, and energy. In low perfusion states where oxygen is not present, the pyruvic acid is not degraded. The pyruvic acid collects and degrades into lactic acid. The accumulation of lactic acid and other metabolic acids results in cellular death. Cellular death leads to tissue death, and tissue death leads to organ death, organ death leads to system death, and system death leads to the death of the patient. *(1.8.1)*

85.

B. The movement and utilization of oxygen is dependent upon factors that make up what is called the "Fick Principle." The factors are: adequate oxygen in the inspired air, oxygen "loaded" on red blood cells, adequate tissue perfusion, and oxygen "off-load" at the body tissues. The three factors required for adequate tissue perfusion are: functioning pump, adequate fluid levels, and an intact container. All three must be working appropriately to produce adequate perfusion pressures. Failure of any one will result in hypoperfusion. Hypoperfusion will yield inadequate oxygenation of body cells or tissues. *(1.8.4)*

86.

C. It is important to adequately ventilate shock patients in order to reduce the acidotic state. Lactic acid production results in the accumulation of hydrogen ions. The more hydrogen ions present in a solution the more acidic the solution. Ensuring adequate ventilation reduces the number of hydrogen ions present. While this reduces the total accumulated acids in the patient's body. Make sure the shock patient's ventilations are adequately supported. *(1.8.5)*

87.

B. Peripheral vascular resistance or afterload is reflected by the diastolic blood pressure. As the peripheral vascular resistance increases, the diastolic blood pressure increases. The reverse occurs as well when the peripheral vascular resistance decreases, the diastolic blood pressure decreases. You would expect to see a slight increase in the diastolic blood pressure as the body's compensatory mechanisms adjust to the diminished perfusion. An early reaction during compensated shock is to increase the peripheral vascular resistance. *(1.8.8)*

88.

A. Blood return or what is called preload is decreased with vasodilation. The "container" size is increased with peripheral vasodilatation. If the amount of fluid in the body remains constant, the amount of fluid available to return to the heart is reduced. The container becomes larger than the available fluid. Some conditions that cause peripheral vasodilatation include decompensated shock, anaphylaxis, septic shock, and vasogenic shock. *(1.8.8)*

89.

D. Most of the body's water, 75% to be exact, is contained within the intracellular fluid. The extracellular fluid is divided as follows: 17.5% interstitial fluid and 7.5% is contained within the vascular space. *(1.8.10)*

90.

C. The most abundant cation (positively charged ion) in the extracellular fluid is sodium. Sodium helps to regulate the movement of water within the various body compartments. A high sodium level is referred to as hypernatremia and a low level is called hyponatremia. *(1.8.11)*

91.

B. Proteins provide the major building blocks of the body. Proteins play a major role in the development of amino acids. Proteins are necessary for body growth, development, and repair. They are a major element in the building of hair, blood, skin, nails, and the interior of organs. Many body hormones are proteins as well. *(1.8.12)*

92.

B. Osmosis is the movement of water across a semi-permeable membrane. Water moves from an area of lower solute concentration to an area of higher solute concentration. The movement of solutes across the semi-permeable membrane is called diffusion. Solutes move from an area of greater solute concentration to an area of lesser solute concentration. Diffusion and osmosis occur to balance the solute concentrations on both sides of a semi-permeable membrane. *(1.8.13)*

93.

D. A solution that is lower in solute concentration when compared to a solution on the opposite side of a semi-permeable membrane is called a hypotonic solution. If the solute concentration is higher than the solution on the opposite side of the semi-permeable membrane it is called hypertonic. A balanced concentration of solutes on both sides is called an isotonic solution. *(1.8.14)*

94.

C. Potassium is the chief intracellular ion. Potassium plays an important role in the transmission of electrical impulses. Low levels of potassium is called hypokalemia and high levels is called hyperkalemia. *(1.8.17)*

95.

B. The statement best describes acid-base balance. The more hydrogen ions present in a solution, the more acidic the solution. The fewer hydrogen ions present in a solution, the more basic or alkaline the solution. This balance is constantly changing in relationship to alterations in body physiology. *(1.8.18)*

96.

D. A pH less than 7.35 is consider acidotic. A pH of greater then 7.45 is considered alkalotic. The normal body pH range is 7.35 to 7.45. The lower the pH, the greater the concentration of hydrogen ions. The higher the pH, the lower the concentration of hydrogen ions. *(1.8.19)*

97.

A. When a patient is hypoventilating, carbon dioxide is retained. The retention of carbon dioxide increases carbonic acid concentration. When the carbonic acid concentration increases, more hydrogen ions are released and the pH value falls. *(1.8.20a)*

98.

B. Hyperventilation results in increased amounts of carbon dioxide being removed or blown off. This reduces the total number of hydrogen ions present. The decrease in the hydrogen ion concentration increases the pH level. This is called respiratory alkalosis. *(1.8.20b)*

99.

C. During low perfusion states, anaerobic metabolism produces lactic acid. The lactic acid releases hydrogen ions which lowers the pH. This is called metabolic acidosis. *(1.8.20c)*

100.

D. The ingestion of antacids or excessive vomiting increases the bicarbonate ions in the blood. This increase in bicarbonate causes the pH value to increase. An increase above 7.45 is termed metabolic alkalosis. *(1.8.20d)*

101.

B. Restlessness or anxiety is an early sign of cerebral hypoxia. This is a result of diminished perfusion and oxygenation of cerebral tissue. An alteration in the patient's level of consciousness, disorientation, and confusion are signs of cerebral hypoperfusion and hypercapnea. *(1.8.27)*

102.

C. Signs of decompensated shock would include an increase in the pulse rate and a decrease in the pulse amplitude. A falling systolic blood pressure is a late sign that is observed in decompensated shock. The skin color would be pale or cyanotic, cool, and moist. The pulse pressure will become more narrow as the condition progresses. *(1.8.28)*

103.

C. Absolute contraindications for the use of the PASG include pulmonary edema and penetrating injuries to the chest and/or neck. Relative contraindications include late pregnancy, impaled object in the abdomen, and head injuries. *(1.8.31)*

104.

D. Lactated Ringer's, normal saline, and 5% dextrose in water are all considered crystalloids. Lactated Ringer's solution and normal saline stay in the intravascular compartment longer than does 5% dextrose in water. Normal saline and lactated Ringer's solution will stay in the vascular space for up to one hour before moving into the interstitial space. Colloids such as plasmanate, albumin, dextran, and hetastarch contain proteins or large glucose molecules. Because of the high molecular weight, they tend to stay in the vascular space for long time periods. *(1.8.32)*

105.

A. Lactated Ringer's solution is the preferred solution to use for the trauma patient that requires volume replacement. Normal saline is also an acceptable solution to use. Dextran and hespan are both colloid solutions. Colloid solutions are not used as often in prehospital care because of problems associated with storage and expense. *(1.8.32)*

106.

D. During fluid replacement therapy, it is important to monitor the patient's pulse, blood pressure, skin temperature, and color. Auscultate the chest frequently. Observe for signs of fluid overload such as dyspnea, pulmonary congestion (edema), and altered mental status. *(1.8.33)*

107.

C. This patient is exhibiting signs of a transfusion reaction. This occurs from the administration of blood or blood products. Additional signs and symptoms include hypotension, fever, chills, tachycardia, flushing of the skin, headaches, loss of consciousness, vomiting, and shortness of breath. *(1.8.33)*

108.

C. The intravenous route is most commonly used for fluid replacement. The oral route is not used because of problems associated with aspiration. There is also a delay associated with movement of fluid from the digestive tract to the intravascular system when using the oral route. The intraosseous route is used for children but not used as frequently as the intravenous route. *(1.8.34)*

109.

D. The two most important factors that affect flow rate are the length and diameter of the intravenous catheter. For the patient that requires fluid replacement, use the largest diameter intravenous catheter practical and one of the shortest length. Use the shortest length administration set as well. *(1.8.34)*

110.

D. The largest concentration of body water is in the intracellular compartment; it constitutes 40% of the total body weight. The other major compartment is the extracellular fluid, which comprises only 20%. Interstitial and intravascular fluid is a subcategory of extracellular fluid. *(1.8.10)*

111.

A. The movement of water from space to space is known as osmosis. This is defined as the movement of water from an area of lower solute concentration to higher solute concentration. Diffusion, active transport, and mediated transport all refer to types of movement for formed elements (electrolytes, proteins, etc.). *(1.8.13)*

112.

C. 0.9% sodium chloride is considered to be isotonic with the body so a solution which is 3% sodium chloride is hypertonic. It will draw water into the vascular space. Finally, 0.45% is hypotonic and will result in water exiting from the vascular space. *(1.8.14)*

113.

B. Osmosis is the movement of water from an area of lower solute concentration to one of higher solute concentration. *(1.8.17)*

114.

B. Diffusion is the principle which explains how electrolytes move from an area of high concentration to low concentration in order to provide equalization across a semi-permeable membrane. Active transport and mediated transport is the movement of a substance across a membrane, but it may not be down a gradient. Osmosis is the movement of water only. *(1.8.15)*

115.

A. Sodium requires active transport and is facilitated by the Na^+-K^+ pump. Active transport is a process by which energy is expended in order to move electrolytes across a semi-permeable membrane, against its concentration gradient. *(1.8.16)*

116.

D. Proteins are a basic building block for the body and their roles are numerous. These include influencing fluid tonicity (albumin), in the immune system (antibody formation), and antigens (which influence human blood type). *(1.8.12)*

117.

C. Electrolytes are moved by all methods except forced movement, which is actually a fabricated term. The fluid portion of the body, water, is moved by osmosis. *(1.8.10)*

118.

C. A patient presenting with severe vomiting will lose-HCl acid from the gastric secretions causing an increase in the bicarbonate ions in the blood. In severe cases the bicarbonate ions will cause metabolic alkalosis. *(1.8.20d)*

119.

D. Persons not acclimated to high elevations tend to have an increased respiratory rate due to the lower levels of oxygen. This increases alveolar ventilation resulting in more CO_2 excretion with exhalation. *(1.8.20b)*

120.

B. Proteins are generally larger molecules which cannot cross the semi-permeable membranes easily. As such, they tend to stay in their original location and because they are a larger molecule, they exert oncotic pressure that keeps water within that particular space. *(1.8.12)*

121.

C. Carbon dioxide is eliminated from the body by exhalation. If a medical or traumatic condition causes reduction in alveolar ventilation, then carbon dioxide levels will continue to rise until they develop respiratory acidosis. Respiratory acidosis is a $PaCO_2$ level greater than 45 mmHg. *(1.8.20a)*

122.

D. The blood buffer system is the first to respond to hydrogen change. And according to the equation for hydrogen buffering, drops in hydrogen ion concen-

tration will cause less conversion to carbonic acid, and diminished CO_2 levels. This is because there is less carbonic acid to dissociate into carbon dioxide and water. *(1.8.19)*

123.

B. Compensation for metabolic acidosis will cause an increase in respiratory rate and depth in an attempt to reduce the CO_2 level and carbonic acid level, causing an increase in the pH. *(1.8.20b)*

124.

B. Metabolic alkalosis means there is a marked decrease in hydrogen ion concentration (pH greater than 7.45). In order to increase hydrogen ion concentration, the kidneys will retain more hydrogen (but this is a slow response), and the respiratory rate will slow so that more CO_2 can be retained and converted back into hydrogen (this is an immediate response). *(1.8.19)*

125.

D. Anaerobic metabolism occurs when there is a lack of sufficient oxygen for cellular metabolism. This leads to production of lactic acid. Failure of the sodium/potassium pump from hypoxemia cause cells to rupture and liberation of lysosome. *(1.8.1)*

126.

C. There are three clinical stages of shock: compensatory, decompensatory, and irreversible. This patient is exhibiting signs of the first stage. *(1.8.24)*

127.

B. During distributive shock there is profound peripheral vasodilitation causing blood pooling in the extremities and promoting hypotension. This will decrease the amount of blood returning to the heart, causing a diminished preload. The decreased preload will decrease cardiac output and blood pressure. *(1.8.9)*

128.

D. Anaerobic metabolism occurs when there is an insufficient supply of oxygen available to meet the demands of the tissues. Constantly ensure the patient is receiving an appropriate amount of oxygen (increase FiO_2, or the fraction of inspired oxygen). *(1.8.2)*

129.

C. The radial pulse and systolic blood pressure are used to guide fluid administration. The goal is to establish a radial pulse and/or a systolic blood pressure of 90 mmHg. *(1.8.32)*

130.

A. When providing fluid replacement for blood loss, infuse at a wide-open rate at increments of 20 ml/kg. If the patient is still showing clinical signs of shock and has no radial pulse or the systolic blood pressure is less than 90 mmHg, repeat the 20 ml/kg bolus and again reassess. *(1.8.33)*

131.

C. The PASG will increase the afterload. Thus, in a patient with pump failure, the further increase in resistance may cause the left ventricle to fail faster. *(1.8.31)*

132.

D. This patient will most likely suffer hypoxia and hypercapnia because of the flail segment. Oxygen levels will continue to diminish with poor ventilations, and carbon dioxide levels will continue to rise. *(1.8.5)*

133.

A. During shock, the brain is also affected by hypoperfusion. The best indicator of poor cerebral perfusion is decreased mental status. Pupillary response will usually be altered also by hypoperfusion, but it is not as reliable as the level of consciousness. *(1.8.27)*

134.

C. 5% dextrose in water is a solution which contains glucose in sterile water. It is prepared as an isotonic solution, but upon administration the glucose is rapidly metabolized, leaving nothing but free water (which is hypotonic). The result is volume leaving the vascular space. As such, this solution will not increase intravascular volume any appreciable amount. *(1.8.32)*

135.

D. Inspiratory crackle is an early indication that the body may be receiving too much fluid. So the IV rate needs to be cut back, but not stopped, in case the IV route is needed for another purpose. A repeat of the bolus could precipitate pulmonary edema, and initiating another IV is unnecessary if the patient has received enough fluid already. *(1.8.33)*

136.

C. In a hypovolemic patient the goal is intravenous cannulation that will allow rapid fluid infusion if needed. The arrangement of a 16-gauge angio with a macrodrip administration set will allow the fastest flow rate. The 14-gauge response is an appropriate gauge for trauma, but the microdrip administration set would be prohibitive if infusing fluids rapidly. *(1.8.34)*

137.

A. Starling's Law discusses the increase in myocardial contraction when the muscle fibers are stretched by increases in preload. The enhanced recoil results in more forceful expulsion of a larger amount of blood. This increase in stroke volume will then translate into improved cardiac output and eventually as improved blood pressure. *(1.8.6)*

138.

B. The application of the PASG will allow an increase in perfusion pressure primarily by mechanical vasoconstriction with inflation of the air bladders. The increase in afterload can raise blood pressure. By decreasing preload and/or afterload, blood pressure will certainly decrease. *(1.8.29)*

139.

C. Baroreceptors are specialized sensors located in the aortic arch and carotid bodies. These unique sensors monitor blood pressure in these arterial blood vessels, and feed this information to the vasomotor center in the medulla. Peripheral chemoreceptors are sensors that monitor oxygen levels, and central chemoreceptors are sensors that monitor hydrogen levels and are located on the medulla. There are no specific receptors for monitoring the heart rate. *(1.8.22)*

140.

D. At the cellular level, the arterial blood will release oxygen to the cells. The high levels of carbon dioxide will then move into the capillary to be transported back to the lungs for elimination. Factors which will increase the release of oxygen into the tissues are elevated temperature, acidic environment, and higher levels of 2,3 DPG. *(1.8.4)*

141.

B. A hypotonic solution is one that has a lower tonicity than that of the body, and the water will leave the vascular space because of osmosis. A hypertonic solution will increase intravascular volume as it pulls excess water in. An isotonic solution will maintain and possibly increase intravascular volume. *(1.8.32)*

142.

D. Of the listed abnormalities, a dehydrated patient is one that needs volume replacement, and lactated Ringer's serves as a isotonic crystalloid which will increase intravascular volume. Cardiac patients and head injury patients usually receive normal saline at a KVO rate, while it is not uncommon for a cardiac patient to receive 5% dextrose in water. *(1.8.34)*

143.

B. An increase in pulmonary capillary hydrostatic pressure will cause fluid to leak out of the capillary and fill the space between the alveoli and the capillary interfering with oxygen and carbon dioxide diffusion. This will eventually lead to hypoxia. *(1.8.3)*

144.

A. As a general rule, oxygen and carbon dioxide will diffuse from areas of high concentration to areas of low concentration. In the alveolar-capillary network, high amounts of oxygen and low amounts of carbon dioxide are found in the alveoli, whereas low amounts of oxygen and higher amounts of carbon dioxide are found in the blood entering the capillary. The gas moves from the higher concentration to lower causing oxygen to enter the blood and carbon dioxide to enter the alveoli. *(1.8.3)*

145.

C. The diastolic blood pressure is a measurement of the systemic vascular resistance. The narrow pulse pressure (systolic minus the diastolic) and pale, cool, clammy skin are indicative of peripheral vasoconstriction which causes an increased systemic vascular resistance. *(1.8.7)*

146.

C. The earliest sign of an increase in systemic vascular resistance is pale, cool, clammy skin. This sign results from a decreased perfusion of peripheral skin and subcutaneous tissue. *(1.8.7)*

147.

D. A decrease in venous volume will directly result in a reduction in the preload or the amount of blood in the left ventricle at the end of diastole. *(1.8.9)*

148.

B. Calcium (CA^{++}) is a cation, which is an ion with a positive charge. Chloride, bicarbonate, and phosphate all have negative charges and are all called anions. *(1.8.11)*

149.

A. Bicarbonate has a negative charge and is an anion in the body. Bicarbonate plays a major role in the blood buffer system and transportation of carbon dioxide in the blood. *(1.8.11)*

150.

C. Large particles and charged particles move more slowly across a semipermeable membrane. Water contains neither charged or large particles, so it would move freely across the membrane. *(1.8.13)*

151.

B. Hypotonic fluids have a reduced osmotic pressure and will leave the vascular space quickly. Hypertonic fluids have a higher osmotic pressure and would draw fluid into the vascular space. Isotonic fluid's osmotic pressure is equal to that of the fluid inside and outside of the semi-permeable membrane and will not cause a fluid shift to occur. *(1.8.14)*

152.

C. Hypertonic fluids have a higher osmotic pressure than the fluid on the outside of the semi-permeable membrane and will draw fluid into the vascular space. *(1.8.14)*

153.

A. Diffusion of the charged particles out of the vascular space will cause a change in the osmotic pressure inside the vessel and will allow the fluid to leave with the electrolytes. *(1.8.15)*

154.

D. The sodium/potassium pump keeps sodium outside the cell and potassium inside of the cell by active transport. This requires energy to function properly. If the pump would fail, sodium would rush into the cell, water would follow because of the osmotic effect, and the cell would rupture. *(1.8.16)*

155.

B. Active transport requires energy to move molecules across a membrane. Molecules can be moved from a low to high concentration. Active transport is usually faster than diffusion and can move larger molecules than diffusion. *(1.8.16)*

156.

C. As carbon dioxide increases in the blood, it combines with water and forms carbonic acid. The increase in carbonic acid causes the pH value to drop, indicating acidosis. *(1.8.18)*

157.

C. A respiratory rate of 6/minute is hypoventilation. This would result in a buildup of carbon dioxide resulting in respiratory acidosis. *(1.8.20)*

158.

D. The PaO_2 of 98 and $PaCO_2$ of 38 reflect normal values. However, the pH of 7.34 is less than the normal value of 7.40. Since the $PaCO_2$ level is normal, the decrease in the pH must result from a metabolic acidosis. *(1.8.20c)*

159.

B. The patient is in hypovolemic shock. Anaerobic metabolism associated with the poor perfusion state causes an increase in lactic acid leading to metabolic acidosis. Because the respiratory rate and depth is relatively normal, it is unlikely the patient has a respiratory acidosis or alkalosis. *(1.8.20c)*

160.

A. Aspirin is salicylic acid, which causes metabolic acidosis when ingested in large quantities. An increase in respiratory rate is an attempt to decrease $PaCO_2$ by blowing off CO_2 and reduce the metabolic acid level. *(1.8.20c)*

161.

A. A patient who continuously vomits over a longer period of time reduces the hydrochloric acid load in the body resulting in metabolic alkalosis. The metabolic alkalosis causes the pH value to increase above 7.40. *(1.8.20d)*

162.

C. An immediate response to a drop in blood pressure causes a direct neural response from the sympathetic nervous system. A nerve fiber stimulates the adrenal medulla to release catecholamines, epinephrine, and norepinephrine. It takes a few minutes for the hormonal response to be activated. *(1.8.21)*

163.

D. A decrease in the blood volume and pressure in the aortic arch and carotid bodies cause a decrease in the stretch of the baroreceptor. The baroreceptor initiates the cascade effect of compensatory mechanisms seen in shock. *(1.8.22)*

164.

B. An increase in the stretch of the baroreceptor indicates an increase in pressure. To reduce the pressure, the body's response will be to reduce heart rate, stroke volume, and peripheral vascular resistance by vasodilation. *(1.8.23)*

165.

B. Pale, cool, clammy skin provides the earliest sign of peripheral vasoconstriction. Since the skin is the most nonessential organ its perfusion is reduced first through peripheral vasoconstriction. The blood is shunted away from the periphery and toward the core circulation. *(1.8.26)*

166.

C. A narrow pulse pressure is the best indication of compensatory shock. The pulse pressure is the difference between the systolic and diastolic blood pressure. A normal pulse pressure is 30 to 40 mmHg. In compensatory shock, the systolic blood pressure decreases due to the decrease in preload, however, the diastolic blood pressure will maintain itself due to the increase in peripheral vascular resistance narrowing the difference between the two readings. *(1.8.28)*

167.

C. The PASG is contraindicated in any patient with intrathoracic trauma and bleeding or isolated head injury with hypotension. The PASG can be used in the patient with a suspected abdominal injury and suspected pelvic fracture. A patient with hemoptysis, bloody sputum, would indicate a lung or respiratory tract injury and this would be a contraindication to application of the PASG. *(1.8.30)*

168.

D. Human serum albumin is a hypertonic solution and will draw fluid into the intravascular space. Lactated Ringer's and normal saline are both isotonic solutions and will not cause a fluid shift. Packed cells will have no osmotic effect. *(1.8.32)*

169.

A. When infusing fluid in elderly patients, it is extremely important to assess frequently for fluid overload. Assess the breath sounds in the lower lobes of the lungs for crackles indicating fluid in the alveoli. If crackles are found, immediately reduce the fluid infusion and monitor the respiratory status and oxygenation of the patient. *(1.8.33)*

170.

B. When infusing fluid in a patient with internal hemorrhage that cannot be controlled, the goal of fluid resuscitation is to infuse only enough fluid to regain a radial pulse or increase the systolic blood pressure to 90 mmHg. More aggressive fluid infusion may cause a more rapid blood loss and is contraindicated. *(1.8.33)*

171.

A. Fluid can be infused at a rate of 20 ml/kg in a patient with blood loss where the bleeding is controlled. If the bleeding is controlled, the systolic blood pressure can be raised above 100 mmHg. *(1.8.33)*

172.

D. The fluid can be infused the most rapidly by using a 14-gauge catheter with a 10-drop macrodrip solution set. *(1.8.34)*

173.

B. A pyrogenic reaction occurs from contaminated fluid, tubing, or catheters. It presents as a sudden onset of fever, chills, headache, nausea, and vomiting. Upon recognition, you should immediately stop and disconnect the IV line. Initiate another IV with a new solution, tubing, and catheter at a new site. *(1.8.34)*

174.

A. Hydrogen ion concentration is inversely proportionate to the pH value. An increase in hydrogen ions will cause the pH value to drop, whereas, a decrease in hydrogen ion concentration will cause the pH value to increase. *(1.8.18)*

9 Defibrillation

chapter objectives

Questions in this chapter relate to DOT objectives 1.9.1–1.9.29. Please see the Appendix for more information.

DIRECTIONS Each of the questions or incomplete statements below is followed by suggested answers or completions. Select the **one answer** that is best in each case.

1. Which of the following best describes the valvular anatomy of the heart?
   A. The pulmonic valve is connected to the right ventricle via the chordae tendonae.
   B. The bicuspid valve is connected to the left atrium via the endocardium.
   C. The aortic valve is connected to the myocardium via the papillary muscle.
   D. The tricuspid valve is connected to the right ventricle via the papillary muscle.

2. Which term best describes the ability of the heart to initiate its own rhythm?
   A. excitability
   B. conductivity
   C. automaticity
   D. contractility

3. A 59-year-old male complains of substernal chest pain that radiates to the left shoulder. Which of the items from his past medical history would be a priority in verbal radio communication with the receiving physician?
   A. kidney stones
   B. high blood pressure
   C. past surgery for appendicitis
   D. dislocated ankle

4. Which of the following signs would suggest that an individual's chest pain may be cardiac in nature?
   A. surgical scar over the sternum
   B. left dilated pupil
   C. jugular venous distention while lying flat
   D. edema of the right hand

5. The purpose of the cardiac conduction system is to initiate an impulse, spread it through the atria, and transmit it:

   A. quickly to the apex of the heart to stimulate ventricular depolarization in an inferior to superior direction.
   B. slowly to the ventricles, stimulating depolarization in a superior to inferior direction to maximize output.
   C. quickly to the intraventricular septum to stimulate depolarization simultaneously in both ventricles from top to bottom.
   D. slowly to the apex of the heart to stimulate each ventricle to depolarize simultaneously by triggering lateral movement.

6. Assessment of the jugular veins should be given special attention in the patient with suspected cardiac problems because:
   A. flat neck veins indicate hypovolemia which may be causing the cardiac malfunction.
   B. neck veins will reflect red blood cell oxygenation and the adequacy of pump action.
   C. the presence of visible pulsatile movement is a sign of a partial obstruction of blood flow.
   D. distention indicates an increase of pressure in the systemic venous circulation due to pump failure.

7. The presence of peripheral edema seen during the physical exam of the cardiac patient indicates:
   A. chronic obesity which is a risk factor for coronary artery disease.
   B. a significant malfunction in the renal system.
   C. congestion in the systemic venous circulation.
   D. a sedentary lifestyle which is a risk factor for coronary artery disease.

8. The heart valve that prevents the regurgitation of blood flow between the right atrium and right ventricle is the:
   A. mitral valve.
   B. semilunar valve.
   C. tricuspid valve.
   D. pulmonic valve.

9. Which vessel delivers blood from venous circulation below the heart and empties into the right atrium?
   A. inferior vena cava
   B. superior vena cava
   C. pulmonary veins
   D. pulmonary arteries

10. Which coronary artery branches off the left coronary artery and supplies oxygenated blood to the left ventricle and the intraventricular septum?
    A. marginal artery
    B. anterior descending
    B. right coronary artery
    C. posterior descending artery

11. Which layer of a blood vessel gives it strength and recoil and is made up of elastic fibers and muscle?
    A. tunica adventia
    B. tunica intima
    C. tunica media
    D. tunica lumen

12. The amount of blood ejected from the right and left ventricles during one contraction is called the:
    A. Starling's Law.
    B. stroke volume.
    C. cardiac output.
    D. cardiac cycle.

13. During the cardiac "action potential" which of the following actions take place?

A. Sodium is pumped out of the cardiac cell membrane by the sodium-potassium pump.
B. Sodium ions rush into the cardiac cells causing them to become positively charged.
C. More negative anions remain inside the cell than the positively charged cations.
D. Potassium leaves the inside of the cell, causing the inside to become negatively charged.

14. Which of the following statements best describes the function of the electrocardiogram (ECG)?
    A. The ECG records the systolic and diastolic pressures.
    B. The ECG records only positive impulses from the heart.
    C. The ECG is a measurement of the heart's pumping ability.
    D. The ECG is a graphic record of the heart's electrical activity.

15. The P wave on an electrocardiogram tracing represents which of the following?
    A. depolarization of the atria
    B. repolarization of the atria
    C. depolarization of the ventricles
    D. repolarization of the ventricles

16. You are analyzing the heart rate on an ECG; your patient has eight complexes within two 3-second marked sections on the ECG graph paper. The heart rate is:
    A. 40 beats per minute.
    B. 60 beats per minute.
    C. 80 beats per minute.
    D. 160 beats per minute.

17. All of the following are dysrhythmias that originate in the atria, **except**:
    A. wandering pacemaker.
    B. premature atrial contractions.

C. supraventricular tachycardia.

D. premature ventricular complexes.

18. The valve that prevents back flow into the left ventricle is the:

A. aortic valve.

B. pulmonic valve.

C. mitral valve.

D. tricuspid valve.

19. The AV node is located inferior to the:

A. bundle of His.

B. bundle branches.

C. Purkinje fibers.

D. SA node.

20. The "P" of the PQRST mnemonic used for assessing chest pain stands for:

A. pain.

B. palliation.

C. past medical history.

D. prescriptions.

21. An ECG complex that covers three small boxes represents:

A. 0.04 seconds.

B. 0.12 seconds.

C. 0.20 seconds.

D. 0.60 seconds.

22. What anatomic structure is incorrectly paired with a physical description?

A. tricuspid valve—separates the right atrium and the right ventricle

B. pulmonary artery—receives blood from the right ventricle

C. left coronary artery—anterior descending and circumflex artery

D. papillary muscle—separates the walls of the ventricles

23. Complete this formula: blood pressure = cardiac output ¥ _____.

A. heart rate

B. stroke volume

C. peripheral vascular resistance

D. Starling's Law

24. Ventricular filling most depends upon:

A. afterload.

B. preload.

C. pulse rate.

D. blood pressure.

25. A common chief complaint of cardiac patients is chest pain or discomfort. Which of the following is suggestive of the pain associated with an acute myocardial infarction?

A. A change in body position alleviates the pain.

B. The pain is frequently located in the lateral chest.

C. The pain often radiates.

D. A change in body position aggravates the pain.

26. A patient you are caring for describes his heart as "skipping beats" or sometimes like it's "racing rapidly." The term that best describes this patient's sensation is:

A. tachy-brady syndrome.

B. palpitations.

C. chest discomfort.

D. cardiac awareness.

27. A syncopal episode that occurs in a patient with a cardiac history is most commonly the result of:

A. the discomfort associated with the chest pain.

B. dysrhythmias such as bradycardia or tachycardia.

C. electrolyte imbalances resulting from extensive diuretic use.

D. excessive fluid loss from diarrhea or vomiting.

28. Which of the following types of questions is least appropriate to ask a cardiac patient complaining of dyspnea?
    A. How long have you been short of breath?
    B. Did this occur gradually or suddenly?
    C. Does your chest hurt?
    D. Are you having any associated symptoms?

29. Common causes of ECG artifact include all of the following, **except**:
    A. patient movement.
    B. muscle tremor.
    C. radio transmission interference.
    D. low battery.

30. The first negative deflection following the P wave is called the:
    A. Q wave.
    B. R wave.
    C. S wave.
    D. T wave.

31. Acute pulmonary edema could occur with the failure of which cardiac valve?
    A. tricuspid
    B. bicuspid
    C. aortic
    D. pulmonary

32. The portion of the cardiac conduction system which is responsible for slowing the impulse down while the ventricles fill with blood is the:
    A. bundle of His.
    B. sinoatrial node.
    C. bundle branch.
    D. atrioventricular node.

33. A cardiac patient presents with severe pitting edema to the ankles, JVD, and clear breath sounds. This is most consistent with:
    A. atrial fibrillation.
    B. left heart failure.
    C. right heart failure.
    D. failure of the mitral valve.

34. The fibrous sac that protects the heart within the thoracic cavity is known as the:
    A. pericardial sac.
    B. endocardial layer.
    C. pericardial space.
    D. epicardium.

35. Cardiac output is a dynamic relationship between:
    A. heart rate and preload.
    B. afterload and contractility.
    C. stroke volume and preload.
    D. heart rate and stroke volume.

36. An ECG is regular if the distance between _____ is even.
    A. every third QRS complex
    B. P and T waves
    C. R waves
    D. a Q wave and the next S wave

37. You are attempting to analyze an ECG rhythm and determine its rate. You count 15 small boxes (1 mm), or 3 large boxes between two consecutive QRS complexes. The heart rate is:
    A. 300 beats per minute.
    B. 150 beats per minute.
    C. 100 beats per minute.
    D. 75 beats per minute.

38. Coronary artery perfusion occurs during:
    A. ventricular systole.
    B. ventricular filling.
    C. atrial contraction.
    D. ventricular diastole.

39. You are assessing a patient with a chief complaint of chest pain. Which of the following information from the past medical history is most relevant?
   A. allergy to morphine
   B. history of two myocardial infarctions
   C. father died of a heart attack at the age of 48
   D. history of strokes

40. Which one of the following abnormal assessment findings is least consistent with a patient in a cardiac emergency?
   A. unequal pupils
   B. irregular heart rate
   C. high blood pressure
   D. difficulty in breathing

41. Which of the following best describes the anatomic location of the apex of the heart?
   A. inferior to the diaphragm and to the right of the midline
   B. at the level of the second rib and to the left of the sternum
   C. to the left of the midline and superior to the diaphragm
   D. in the retromediastinal space at the inferior costochondral margin

42. Which of the following structures prevents regurgitation of blood back into the left ventricle during ventricular diastole?
   A. tricuspid valve
   B. mitral valve
   C. pulmonic valve
   D. aortic valve

43. Which of the following best describes the epicardium?
   A. It is the outermost lining of the heart that is contiguous with the visceral pericardium.
   B. It is the innermost lining of the atria and ventricles.
   C. It is the bulk of muscle mass that produces the contractile force.
   D. It is the layer that houses the pericardial fluid.

44. Which of the following sentences most accurately defines the chordae tendonae?
   A. They are specialized muscles in the ventricles that open the mitral and tricuspid valves.
   B. They are specialized fibers that connect the leaflets of the mitral and tricuspid valves to the papillary muscles.
   C. It is conduction tissue that is located in the myocardium of the left ventricle.
   D. They are connective fibers that anchor the aortic and pulmonic valves in place.

45. Which of the following are the terminal branches of the conduction system that are responsible for delivering the electrical impulse to the ventricular muscle?
   A. internodal tracts
   B. bundle branches
   C. Purkinje fibers
   D. bundle of His

46. Which of the following ions enter the cardiac cell during depolarization?
   A. sodium and calcium
   B. potassium and sodium
   C. potassium and calcium
   D. sodium only

47. Which of the following would accurately depict atrial repolarization on an ECG tracing?
   A. P wave
   B. Q wave
   C. QRS complex
   D. T wave

48. Which of the following signs or symptoms would best represent transient symptomatic bradycardia in an elderly patient?
    A. diarrhea
    B. headache
    C. nausea and vomiting
    D. syncope

49. You are treating a patient with chest pain when suddenly the monitor shows what appears to be a chaotic and disorganized rhythm with varying amplitudes and no discernable waves or complexes. The patient continues to complain of worsening chest pain and dyspnea. You should immediately:
    A. defibrillate at 200 joules.
    B. check the carotid pulse.
    C. check the electrodes and wires.
    D. begin chest compressions.

50. If you wanted to determine the patient's heart rate by counting the number of complexes in a 6-second strip, how many large boxes on the ECG grid paper would you count to arrive at 6 seconds?
    A. 60
    B. 30
    C. 15
    D. 2

51. An AED should **not** be immediately applied to a patient who:
    A. has an automated implanted cardiac defibrillator.
    B. has a history of open heart surgery.
    C. has suffered a traumatic cardiac arrest.
    D. is pulseless but severely diaphoretic.

52. The AED should only be applied to a patient who is:
    A. younger than 12 years of age
    B. older than 18 years of age
    C. younger than 16 years of age
    D. older than 8 years of age

53. The most common source of inappropriate shocks while using the AED results from:
    A. inappropriate rhythm analysis.
    B. operator error.
    C. cable detachment.
    D. muscular movement.

54. Which of the following represents the most critical factor associated with successful resuscitation when using the AED?
    A. time to defibrillation
    B. bystander CPR
    C. ability to administer antiarrhythmic drugs
    D. immediate transport capabilities

55. What is the most common initial rhythm the patient will present with in sudden cardiac death?
    A. asystole
    B. supraventricular tachycardia
    C. pulseless electrical activity
    D. ventricular fibrillation

56. When using the AED, CPR should be interrupted:
    A. for no more than 15 seconds.
    B. for less than 30 seconds.
    C. long enough for the three stacked shocks to be delivered.
    D. only during the analysis period and after the first set of stacked shocks.

57. When the AED is in the analysis mode, you must:
    A. stop chest compressions but continue to ventilate.
    B. keep your fingers on the carotid artery to check for return of a spontaneous pulse.
    C. stop CPR and ventilation and stand clear of the patient.

D. call for ALS backup, connect the oxygen to the reservoir, and insert an oropharyngeal airway.

58. The AED indicates a shock. Immediately prior to pressing the shock button, you must:

A. check the patient's pulse and breathing.

B. ensure that everyone is clear of the patient.

C. check the cable and lead placement.

D. verify the rhythm on the oscilloscope.

59. You have resuscitated the patient prior to transport. While en route to the hospital, your patient suddenly becomes unresponsive. You should immediately

A. stop the ambulance, turn the engine off, and press the analyze button.

B. check the patient's pulse and breathing.

C. immediately press the analyze button.

D. begin CPR and continue transport.

60. You have delivered two shocks to the patient. After the second shock, the AED indicates a "no shock advisory." You should immediately

A. check the pulse and breathing.

B. press the analyze button.

C. charge the defibrillator for the next shock.

D. begin CPR.

61. You arrive on the scene and find a pulseless and apneic patient. You attach the AED while CPR is in progress. You stop CPR and analyze the rhythm. The AED indicates to "check patient." No pulse or breathing is present. You should next:

A. press the analyze button again, then begin CPR for one minute.

B. perform CPR for one minute, check pulse and breathing, and reanalyze the rhythm.

C. remove the AED and prepare the patient for transport.

D. perform CPR and wait for ALS backup for any further intervention.

62. You arrive on the scene and find a patient on the ground. A family member is performing CPR. You should:

A. have the person continue CPR while you attach the AED.

B. stop the CPR and assess for pulse and breathing.

C. stop CPR and attach the AED.

D. begin bag-valve-mask ventilation with supplemental oxygen.

63. You arrive on the scene and find an adult patient who weighs approximately 75 lbs. He is pulseless and apneic. Your partner begins CPR. You should:

A. proceed with the AED attachment.

B. contact medical direction for permission to attach the AED.

C. continue with CPR only and transport.

D. wait for the ALS backup for defibrillation.

64. The monophasic defibrillation pads should be placed:

A. white to the right of the sternum, red on the left anterior axillary line at the apex.

B. red to the right of the sternum, white on the left anterior axillary line at the apex.

C. white to the left of the sternum, red on the right anterior axillary line at the apex.

D. red to the left of the sternum, white on the right anterior axillary line at the apex.

65. The operator shift checklist should be completed:

A. monthly.

B. weekly.

C. daily.

D. when the low battery light is illuminated.

66. You arrive on the scene and find a 52-year-old male pulseless and apneic. The most important intervention is to:
    A. assist ventilation.
    B. call for ALS backup.
    C. begin CPR for one minute.
    D. apply the AED to the patient.

67. When using a monophasic AED, the first shock is delivered at:
    A. 100 joules.
    B. 200 joules.
    C. 300 joules.
    D. 360 joules.

68. All of the following are components of the "Chain of Survival" **except**:
    A. early ACLS.
    B. bystander CPR.
    C. medical control.
    D. rapid notification of EMS.

69. After delivering the first shock in the series of three shocks to your patient, you must:
    A. begin CPR.
    B. check the pulse.
    C. reanalyze the rhythm.
    D. assist the respirations.

70. You are treating a 67-year-old male complaining of chest pain and difficulty breathing. En route to the hospital he becomes pulseless and apneic. After the second shock, the AED advises "no shock." You should immediately
    A. check pulse and breathing.
    B. check leads and reanalyze.
    C. open the airway and give two breaths.
    D. begin CPR and assist ventilations.

71. Normal electrical conduction of the heart originates in the:
    A. SA node.
    B. AV node.

C. Purkinje fibers.
    D. intra-atrial pathways.

72. You are called to the scene of a near drowning. Your patient has been underwater for approximately 30 minutes and is pulseless and apneic. His core body temperature is 86°F. You should immediately
    A. begin rewarming and transport.
    B. place the AED on the patient and analyze.
    C. start CPR and assist ventilations.
    D. administer 5–10 abdominal thrusts.

73. You and your EMT partner arrive on the scene to find a 63-year-old woman in cardiac arrest. While you are preparing the AED, you should instruct your partner to:
    A. initiate an IV line.
    B. notify medical control.
    C. obtain the past medical history of the patient.
    D. begin CPR and assist ventilation.

74. You arrive on the scene at a local restaurant to find a 34-year-old unresponsive man lying on the floor. His wife states he was talking and suddenly fell to the floor. Your first action should be to:
    A. check pulses and begin CPR.
    B. administer the Heimlich maneuver.
    C. place the AED on the patient and press analyze.
    D. open the airway and attempt to ventilate.

75. After delivering the second shock in the second set of defibrillations, the patient regains a pulse. You should:
    A. remove the AED from the patient and check the blood pressure.
    B. analyze the rhythm.
    C. assess the breathing status and blood pressure.
    D. apply a nonrebreather mask.

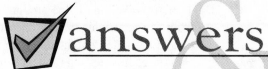
answers & rationales

1.

D. The tricuspid valve separates the right atrium and right ventricle. It is connected to the right ventricle via the papillary muscles and the string-like chordae tendonae. Anatomically speaking, the pulmonic valve and aortic valve function directly off of directional blood flow and do not utilize the chordae tendonae and the papillary muscle structures. Also, similar to the tricuspid valve, the bicuspid valve is manipulated via the papillary muscles and chordae tendonae. These structures then connect to the left ventricle, not the left atrium. *(1.9.2)*

2.

C. Cells of the cardiac conduction system possess the ability of electrical impulse generation without stimulus from an external source. This property is termed automaticity and is responsible for the impulse generation that occurs in the different pacemaking sites of the heart. Excitability and conductivity are electrical properties that pertain to actions that take place after the impulse has been generated. Finally, contractility describes the actions that occur in response to an electrical current or chemical stimulus—not to the origination. *(1.9.7)*

3.

B. High blood pressure directly relates to the cardiovascular system and is therefore a priority in communication to the receiving physician. While the other items should be documented and eventually communicated in this patient, items that directly relate to the cardiac and pulmonary systems take priority. *(1.9.16)*

4.

A. A midsternal scar suggests thoracic surgery, possibly for a previous coronary artery bypass. Isolated pupillary dilation serves little link to cardiac difficulties and jugular venous distention (JVD) upon supination is not uncommon. JVD has a greater significance when present in the seated or standing individual. Cardiac related edema tends to occur in the dependent areas of the body such as the legs. *(1.9.17)*

5.

A. The role of the cardiac conduction system is to stimulate the ventricles to depolarize in an inferior to superior direction, thus maximizing cardiac output. The purpose is to initiate an impulse, spread it through the atria, and transmit it quickly to the apex of the heart to stimulate ventricular depolarization. *(1.9.8)*

6.

D. Jugular vein distention, when seated or standing, indicates an increase in pressure in the systemic venous circulation caused by acute or chronic pump failure. When performing a physical examination on a patient with suspected cardiac problems, special attention should be given to the cardiovascular and respiratory systems. *(1.9.17)*

7.

C. The presence and severity of peripheral edema seen during the physical exam of the cardiac patient indicates congestion in the systemic venous circulation. This can be a sign of acute or chronic pump failure. Assessment of the cardiac patient should be focused on those signs which provide information on the adequacy of cardiac function. *(1.9.18)*

8.

C. The tricuspid valve separates the right atrium from the right ventricle. The tricuspid valve is made up of three distinct leaflets. The mitral valve separates the left atrium from the left ventricle and consists of two leaflets. The semilunar valves are located between the ventricles and arteries they supply. *(1.9.2a)*

9.

A. The inferior vena cava is the large vein that delivers deoxygenated blood from the lower portion of the body. The inferior vena cava empties blood into the right atrium. The superior vena cava is the large vein that delivers deoxygenated blood from the upper body and it empties into the right atrium. The pulmonary vein delivers oxygenated blood from the lungs into the left atrium, and the pulmonary artery carries deoxygenated blood away from the heart (right ventricle) to the lungs. *(1.9.2b)*

10.

B. The anterior descending coronary artery as well as the circumflex coronary artery branch from the left coronary artery. The anterior descending feeds the intraventricular septum. The circumflex feeds the left atrium, left ventricle, and posterior of the right atrium. *(1.9.4)*

11.

C. The tunica media is the middle layer and is made up of muscle and elastic fibers that give the vessel its strength and recoil. The tunica media is much thicker in arteries than veins. The tunica adventitia is the outermost structure and provides strength to withstand the pressure exerted by the contraction of the heart. The tunica intima is the innermost lining of the blood vessel and is a single layer thick. The lumen is the cavity inside the vessel. *(1.9.5)*

12.

B. The stroke volume is the amount of blood ejected from the ventricles during one contraction. Starling's Law states that the more the myocardial muscle is stretched (up to a limit) the greater its force of contraction. Cardiac output is the volume of blood in milliliters pumped by the heart in one minute. It can be calculated with the formula: stroke volume ¥ heart rate = cardiac output. Cardiac cycle is the period from the end of one heart contraction until the end of the next one. *(1.9.6)*

13.

B. During the action potential phase, sodium rushes into the cell bringing a positive charge. This charge is so strong it causes the normal negative resting potential to disappear. This is the start of the depolarization process, leading to muscle contraction. *(1.9.10)*

14.

D. The ECG is a graphic recording of the electrical activity in the heart. This electrical activity is recorded in positive and negative deflections. The ECG does not measure the blood pressure, or heart's pumping ability. It is possible to have a normal electrical impulse on the ECG and have no palpable pulse. *(1.9.11)*

15.

A. The P wave is the first positive deflection, precedes the QRS complex, and represents depolarization of the atria. Repolarization of the atria cannot be seen on the ECG because it is covered by the QRS complex. The QRS complex represents the depolarization of the ventricles. The T wave represents the repolarization of the ventricles. *(1.9.12)*

16.

C. The correct rate is 80 beats per minute and is calculated as follows. Find two 3-second sections and count the number of complexes in the 6-second period, multiply the number of complexes by 10 and you have the answer. *(1.9.22)*

17.

D. Premature ventricular complexes originate in the ventricles. The others originate in the atria. Supraventricular tachycardia sounds like it refers to the ventricles; however, it is *supra-*, meaning above, and *ventricular,* meaning ventricles. Combine the two and you have "above the ventricles." *(1.9.23)*

18.

A. The aortic valve separates the left ventricle from the aorta, preventing back flow into the left ventricle after contraction. The pulmonic valve separates the right ventricle from the pulmonary artery. The mitral valve is between the left atrium and the left ventricle. The tricuspid valve separates the right atrium from the right ventricle. *(1.9.2)*

19.

D. The AV node sits inferior to the SA node at the junction of the right atrium and right ventricle. It is superior to the bundle of His, the bundle branches, and the Purkinje fibers. *(1.9.9)*

20.

D. The "P" of the PQRST mnemonic stands for both provocation and palliation, meaning aggravates or alleviates pain. The "Q" stands for the quality of the pain. The "R" in the mnemonic should trigger the words region, radiation, and recurrence. The "S" stands for severity. The "T" should prompt the EMT-Intermediate to determine the time elements of the chest pain. These are all important questions that need to be asked of any patient experiencing chest pain. *(1.9.15)*

21.

B. Each small box on the ECG paper represents 0.04 seconds. Consequently, three boxes will measure 0.12 seconds. The large boxes, containing 5 small boxes, represents 0.20 seconds. *(1.9.19)*

22.

D. The papillary muscle is a specialized muscle that attaches to the chordae tendonae. The chordae tendonae attaches to the leaflets of the arterioventricular valves and prevents them from prolapsing into the atria during ventricular contraction. *(1.9.2)*

23.

C. Systemic blood pressure is equal to the cardiac output times the peripheral vascular resistance. If either the cardiac output or the peripheral vascular resistance changes and the other item remains constant, the blood pressure will rise or fall, accordingly. Cardiac output is equal to the stroke volume, the amount of blood ejected from the ventricle during one contraction times the heart rate. *(1.9.6)*

24.

B. Ventricular filling occurs during diastole and is a relatively passive event. Only 25% of blood volume is pumped into the ventricle by the atria. The important factor that affects ventricular filling is preload or the amount of blood that is returned to the heart. A decreased preload will result in a decline in filling pressure and a diminished force of contraction. *(1.9.6)*

25.

C. The best answer is radiation of the pain. Often this pain radiates to the shoulder, neck, or arm. Acute myocardial infarction pain is not generally affected by changes in body position. The pain is frequently located substernally and not in the lateral chest. *(1.9.13)*

26.

B. The patient who has an awareness of his heart rate or rhythm is describing what is called palpitations. This is related to the potential presence of a dysrhythmia. *(1.9.14)*

27.

B. Syncope in the cardiac patient is most commonly associated with dysrhythmias which often include bradycardia or tachycardia. Non-cardiac related syncope may result from electrolyte disturbances or fluid balance problems. *(1.9.14)*

28.

C. This question is considered a closed ended question, a question that requires only a yes or no response. It is best to use open ended questions. Form your questions so that you require the patient to provide a descriptive answer. An example of an appropriate question is: "How do you feel?" This would allow the patient to describe in his or her own way how he or she feels. This also prevents you from suggesting symptoms to the patient. *(1.9.15)*

29.

C. Radio transmission interference has been reported to affect AED operation, although it is not considered a common cause of ECG artifact. Additional causes of poor tracings include broken patient cable, broken lead wire, and faulty grounding. *(1.9.20)*

30.

A. The first component of the normal ECG is the P wave. The P wave represents atrial depolarization. The first negative wave that follows the P wave is called the Q wave. The Q wave is part of the QRS complex which represents ventricular depolarization. *(1.9.21)*

31.

B. The bicuspid (or mitral) valve is located between the left atrium and ventricle. Since the left side of the heart is the high-pressure side, the mitral valve is most likely to fail from fatigue. And when it does, blood regurgitates into the atria, which then causes an increase in hydrostatic pressure in the pulmonary capillaries with resultant pulmonary edema. *(1.9.2)*

32.

D. The AV node is the portion of the conduction system that slows the impulse down as it travels from the atria to the ventricles. This is necessary so that the ventricles can fill with blood from atrial contraction. The SA node is the primary pacemaker for the heart while the bundle of His and bundle branches help distribute the impulse wave evenly across the ventricular tissue. *(1.9.9)*

33.

C. This is a classic presentation of pure right-sided heart failure. When the right ventricle starts to fail and pump blood inadequately, it will back up into the right atrium and the vena cavae. As central venous pressure rises, the patient may display both JVD and peripheral edema. When the patient has left-sided heart failure, the lungs usually reveal crackles because of the increased fluid in the alveoli from an increase in hydrostatic pressure in the pulmonary capillaries. *(1.9.18)*

34.

A. The pericardial sac is the fibrous structure that houses and protects the heart. The endocardium and epicardium are both layers of the heart, and the pericardial cavity is the space created by the pericardium for the heart to exist in. *(1.9.2)*

35.

D. Heart rate and stroke volume. The stroke volume is the amount of blood expelled with each individual contraction. Preload, contractility, and afterload are variables that influence the stroke volume. *(1.9.6)*

36.

C. When assessing for the regularity of an ECG strip, you should assess the regularity between consecutive R waves of the ventricular contraction. There should be less than a 0.04-second difference between complexes. *(1.9.21)*

37.

C. There are numerous ways to determine the heart rate on the ECG. One common way is to count the number of large boxes between two consecutive R waves and divide it into 300 (300/3 = 100 per minute). Or you could count the number of small boxes and divide that into 1500 (1500/15 = 100 per minute). *(1.9.19)*

38.

D. The coronary arteries are the first arteries to arise off the base of the aorta. But unlike all other arteries, which are perfused during systole, the coronary arteries are perfused during diastole. This is because as the aortic valves open during systole, they cover the coronary arteries. Blood only reaches the arteries when the valve is closed. *(1.9.2)*

39.

B. Since the patient has a history of two MIs, it is important to assess if this presentation is similar to previous heart attacks. The allergy to morphine is important, but morphine is not administered by the EMT-I. The age of death of the father does not necessarily mean your patient will die at a similar age. A history of strokes is evidence of cardiovascular disease, but is not the most important aspect given the patient's presentation at this time. *(1.9.16)*

40.

A. Unequal pupils are most common with strokes and traumatic head injuries. If poor cardiac output occurs due to an MI, pupillary dilation may occur due to poor cerebral perfusion and hypoxemia, but that should affect each pupil equally. However, an irregular heart rate, hypertension, and dyspnea are not uncommon to an MI. *(1.9.13)*

41.

C. The apex, which is the cone-shaped end of the heart, is to the left of the midline and superior to the diaphragm. It is the bottom section of the heart. *(1.9.1)*

42.

D. The aortic valve prevents regurgitation of blood back into the left ventricle during the diastolic phase because it is located between the left ventricle and aorta. The tricuspid valve prevents blood from flowing back up into the right atrium during contraction of the right ventricle. Likewise, the mitral valve prevents blood flow back into the left atrium during contraction of the left ventricle. The pulmonic valve is similar to the aortic valve, it prevents blood flow back into the right ventricle from the pulmonary arteries during diastole. *(1.9.2)*

43.

A. The epicardium is the outermost lining of the heart that is contiguous with the visceral pericardium. The innermost lining is the endocardium and the myocardium is the bulky muscle mass. The pericardial sac surrounds and houses the pericardial fluid. *(1.9.2)*

44.

B. The chordae tendonae are specialized fibers that connect the leaflets of the mitral and tricuspid valves to the papillary muscles. *(1.9.3)*

45.

C. The terminal segment of the conduction system within the heart is the Purkinje fiber network. This network extends into the ventricular muscle and is responsible for sending the electrical impulse through the bulk of ventricular muscle causing depolarization of the cells and contraction. The bundle of His and bundle branches are also found in the ventricles; however, they are not the terminal branches of the conduction system. *(1.9.9)*

46.

A. During cellular depolarization, sodium rushes into the cell as potassium moves out. Calcium also moves through a slow channel into the cell. The combination is what creates the changes in polarization resulting in muscle contraction. *(1.9.10)*

47.

C. Repolarization of the atria are not represented on the ECG by a specific wave or complex; however, you will find repolarization occurring during the same time the ventricles depolarize. The repolarization of the atria is hidden in the QRS complex which represents depolarization of the ventricles. *(1.9.12)*

48.

D. Syncope may not be a common fainting spell in some patients and needs to be taken seriously. In many elderly patients, syncope is a sign of cardiac dysrhythmias. *(1.9.14)*

49.

C. What is described on the monitor sounds like ventricular fibrillation, however, the patient continues to complain of chest pain and dyspnea indicating he still has pulses and is responsive. This rules out the possibility of ventricular fibrillation. Do not immediately defibrillate your patient until you have checked pulses, breathing, and responsiveness in the patient. If the patient has a pulse with a rhythm that looks similar to ventricular fibrillation, it is probably artifact from a loose electrode. *(1.9.20)*

50.

B. Each large grid box on the ECG paper is 0.2 seconds. Each small box is 0.04 seconds. Therefore, to get a 6-second strip it would be necessary to count 30 large boxes. *(1.9.22)*

51.

C. The primary indication for application of the AED is for cardiac arrest of a medical etiology. In the trauma patient, the most likely etiology of cardiac arrest is due to blunt or penetrating trauma to the myocardium, excessive hypovolemia, head injury, or spinal injury, with a typical presenting rhythm of pulseless electrical activity, asystole, or agonal beats. In the medical patient, the most likely cause of cardiac arrest is a dysrhythmia secondary to coronary artery disease and myocardial ischemia. The presenting rhythm is typically ventricular fib-

rillation. The purpose of the AED is to depolarize fibrillating myocardial tissue to restore a rhythm and cardiac output. In the trauma patient, the rhythm typically does not warrant AED since it is most likely a non-shockable rhythm. Once you have initially managed the trauma patient's airway, breathing, and major life threats and you have provided spinal immobilization and prepared him for transport, consideration can be made to apply the AED. Contact medical direction or follow your local protocol in use of the AED in trauma patients.

52.

D. The use of the AED is appropriate in patients who are eight years of age or older, with an approximate body weight of greater than 25 kg. The use of the AED in infants and children younger than eight years of age is not recommended.

53.

B. The AED is a sophisticated piece of technology that has proven its effectiveness and efficiency in providing defibrillation to patients in cardiac arrest. The most common source of inappropriate functioning, which is extremely rare, is primarily due to operator error. A major error is application of the AED to a patient who has a pulse. The AED should only be applied to pulseless and apneic patients. Failures with AED itself have been associated with the device not delivering a shock when appropriate. Radio transmitters and receivers may interfere with the signals during the analysis phase. Do not transmit over the radio during analysis of the rhythm. Implanted automatic defibrillators may also interfere with the AEDs analysis of the rhythm.

54.

A. The most critical factor associated with successful resuscitation of a patient in cardiac arrest with the aid of automated external defibrillation is time. Early defibrillation is critical to increasing the survival of out-of-hospital cardiac arrest patients. Early defibrillation is paramount to improving chances of a successful resuscitation because the most frequent presenting initial rhythm is ventricular fibrillation. The most effective method to abolish ventricular fibrillation is defibrillation. The sooner the defibrillation is delivered, the better the chance of successful conversion. With each minute that passes, the success rate of defibrillation decreases by about 10%. After a few minutes following cardiac arrest, the rhythm has a tendency to deteriorate to asystole. Thus, the sooner the defibrillation can be delivered, the better the chance of survival for the patient.

55.

D. Ventricular fibrillation is the most common rhythm the patient will present with following cardiac arrest. After a few minutes, the ventricular fibrillation has a tendency to deteriorate to asystole.

56.

C. CPR should be interrupted long enough to deliver the first set of three stacked shocks. This may take up to 90 seconds, during which no CPR is in progress. This is an acceptable delay since the AED has the most beneficial effect in converting the rhythm.

57.

C. During the analysis mode, all contact with the patient must be stopped. Thus, no chest compressions, ventilation, or any other physical contact can be made with the patient. Also, do not transmit on the portable radio during the analysis phase.

58.

B. It is the operator's responsibility to ensure that everyone, including bystanders, are clear of the patient prior to depressing the shock button. There should be absolutely no contact with the patient during both the analysis phase and shock delivery phase.

59.

B. Even with the AED attached, it is necessary that you confirm that the patient is pulseless and apneic prior to initiating analysis of the rhythm.

60.

A. A "no shock indicated" message typically means one of two things: 1) the patient regained a perfusing rhythm with a pulse or 2) the patient has deteriorated to a non-shockable rhythm with no pulse. After any "no shock advisory" or "no shock indicated," the patient's pulse and breathing must be assessed to determine the need for continued CPR or further assessment.

61.

B. After getting a "no shock indicated" message, you must initially assess the pulse and breathing. If no pulse or breathing is present, one minute of CPR is to be performed followed by another analysis of the rhythm. CPR is performed for one minute after each "no shock indicated" message. After three "no shock indicated" messages, it is necessary to prepare the patient for transport.

62.

B. If bystanders or first responders are performing CPR upon your arrival, the first step you should perform is to ensure the patient is still pulseless and apneic. Therefore, stop the CPR and assess the pulse and breathing.

63.

A. An adult patient who weighs 75 pounds can be defibrillated using the standard AED. Biphasic waveform defibrillators deliver energy at lower settings and may prove more effective than the monophasic type.

64.

A. The standard defibrillation pad placement is the white lead electrode pad to the right of the sternum and the red electrode pad to the left apex on the anterior axillary line.

65.

C. The operator shift checklist must be completed for every shift, minimally every day.

66.

D. The AED should be applied as early as possible. Time is the critical element to successful defibrillation. It is more important to defibrillate than to perform CPR, insert airways, or initiate intravenous infusions.

67.

B. The monophasic AED delivers the first defibrillation at 200 joules. The second defibrillation is usually at 300 joules followed by the third defibrillation at 360 joules.

68.

C. Medical direction is a necessary component of the emergency medical services system; however, it is not a true component of the "Chain of Survival."

69.

C. After the first and second shocks in the series of three stacked shocks, the rhythm must be reanalyzed. The older AEDs may require the operator to actually depress a button to reanalyze the rhythm after each shock. The newer models automatically reanalyze the rhythm.

70.

A. After any "no shock indicated" you should immediately assess the pulse and breathing. If the patient has no pulse and is not breathing, begin CPR. If a pulse is present, determine the need to continue to deliver ventilations, and assess the vital signs.

71.

A. The sinoatrial (SA) node is the primary pacemaker of the heart. This is where the electrical impulse that generates a rhythm and cardiac contraction originates.

72.

B. In the hypothermic patient it is appropriate to apply the AED if the patient is determined to be pulseless and apneic. Be sure to assess the pulses in the hypothermic patient for approximately 30 to 45 seconds to be sure that the pulse is not present. If not present, apply the AED and deliver one set of stacked shocks. If this is not successful, do not proceed with any other defibrillation attempts until the patient is adequately rewarmed. This can only be achieved in the hospital.

73.

D. If there will be any delay in preparing the AED for application, have your partner, first responders, or bystanders continue with CPR. As soon as the AED is applied and ready, immediately stop CPR, have everyone clear the patient, and begin with rhythm analysis.

74.

D. You must first establish unresponsiveness, followed by opening the airway and assessing for breathing. If no breathing is present, deliver two ventilations and assess for a pulse. If no pulse is present, apply the AED.

75.

C. If the patient regains a pulse following defibrillation, your next action is to assess the breathing, ventilate if necessary, and take a set of vital signs.

10 Anaphylaxis and Management

chapter objectives

The questions in this chapter serve as a supplement to the curriculum and have no direct relation to the DOT objectives.

DIRECTIONS Each of the questions or incomplete statements below is followed by suggested answers or completions. Select the **one answer** that is best in each case.

1. When a foreign substance is introduced into the bloodstream, the body responds by manufacturing:
   A. antibodies.
   B. antigens.
   C. histamine.
   D. allergens.

2. Sensitization refers to:
   A. the process of creating antigens in response to antibodies.
   B. the release of chemical mediators into the bloodstream.
   C. the body's response to the released chemical mediators.
   D. the body's ability to attack a foreign substance upon repeated exposure.

3. After being manufactured, antibodies can attach themselves to:
   A. esinophils.
   B. basophils.
   C. neutrophils.
   D. monophils.

4. Antibodies are manufactured to eliminate or destroy _____, which may invade the body.
   A. immunoglobulins
   B. haptens
   C. basophils
   D. allergens

5. An anaphylactic reaction can best be described as an:
   A. antibody–hapten reaction.
   B. allergy–antigen reaction.

   C. antigen–antibody reaction.
   D. antigen–allergen reaction.

6. The body system responsible for the anaphylactic reaction is the:
   A. cardiovascular.
   B. immune.
   C. respiratory.
   D. integumentary.

7. What is the primary cause of death in a patient with a severe anaphylactic reaction?
   A. hypotension
   B. laryngeal edema
   C. tachycardia
   D. bronchospasm

8. Hypotension is seen with a severe anaphylactic reaction caused by:
   A. peripheral shunting of blood.
   B. the antigen introduced into the bloodstream.
   C. vasoconstriction.
   D. a decrease in systemic vascular resistance.

9. Which of the following respiratory assessment findings is not consistent with anaphylaxis?
   A. bronchospasm
   B. decreased airway resistance
   C. increased mucous production
   D. bronchial edema

10. Increased vascular permeability and vasodilation secondary to anaphylaxis causes:
    A. hypotension.
    B. bradycardia.

C. tachypnea.

D. hyperpnea.

11. Urticaria and pruritis associated with anaphylaxis is primarily caused by:

A. chemical mediator release from MAST cells.

B. cellular changes from profound hypoxia.

C. erythemic tissue.

D. acidosis secondary to hypoperfusion.

12. One of the most prevalent chemical mediators associated with an anaphylactic reaction is:

A. phosphodiasterase.

B. cyclic-AMP.

C. histamine.

D. glucagon.

13. An acute anaphylactic reaction could occur after the antigen was _____ into the body.

A. injected

B. ingested

C. inhaled

D. all of the above

14. Which of the following is least likely to cause anaphylaxis?

A. wasp venom

B. certain medications

C. pollen

D. food

15. Basophils are found primarily in:

A. connective tissue.

B. the respiratory tree.

C. vascular smooth muscle.

D. circulating blood.

16. What are the hallmark integumentary signs indicative of an anaphylactic reaction?

A. pruritis and urticaria

B. rhinorrhea and edema

C. erythema and lesions

D. urticaria and rhinorrhea

17. You are assessing a 21-year-old male who was stung by a bee. The patient was initially complaining of hives, itching, wheezing, and tightness in his chest, but now has a diminishing level of consciousness, is extremely cyanotic, and hypotensive. Based on the given signs, he is experiencing which type of anaphylactic reaction?

A. mild

B. moderate

C. severe

D. fatal

18. Bronchoconstriction associated with an anaphylactic reaction is manifested as:

A. stridorous respirations.

B. wheezing upon auscultation.

C. crackles upon auscultation.

D. rhonchi upon auscultation.

19. Which of the following is an ominous sign of impending arrest in a severe anaphylactic reaction?

A. tachycardia above 100 per minute

B. cyanosis to the extremities

C. minimal wheezing with diminished breath sounds upon auscultation

D. loss of radial pulses and a systolic blood pressure of 102 mmHg.

20. How is glottic edema, associated with an anaphylactic reaction, manifested in severe anaphylaxis?

A. wheezing

B. stridor

C. hemoptysis

D. pruritis

21. Respiratory stridor indicates:
    A. bronchoconstriction.
    B. airway occlusion.
    C. massive vasodilation.
    D. hypoperfusion.

22. What vital signs are most consistent with severe anaphylaxis?
    A. BP 100/86, HR 68, RR 18
    B. BP 86/68, HR 130, RR 42
    C. BP 180/90, HR 140, RR 36
    D. BP 78/64, HR 98, RR 18

23. You have assessed and begun treatment on a 36-year-old male suffering an anaphylactic reaction. Initially, the patient was extremely dyspneic with coarse bilateral wheezing, disoriented, cool, clammy skin, and was hypotensive. Currently, the patient is still hypotensive and disoriented, but now the breath sounds have diminished even further. Based on the presented findings, you conclude that:
    A. the patient's status is probably improving.
    B. the patient's status is probably unchanged.
    C. the patient's status is probably deteriorating.
    D. you do not have enough information to tell.

24. As a general guideline, the _____ the onset of signs and symptoms of anaphylaxis after exposure, the severity of the reaction is _____.
    A. quicker, milder
    B. slower, milder
    C. quicker, increased
    D. slower, increased

25. A severe anaphylactic reaction:
    A. can occur with minutes after exposure.
    B. usually occurs within 10 to 15 minutes of exposure.

C. usually develops over 30 minutes after exposure.
D. takes at least an hour to develop after exposure.

26. Physical indications of histamine release in a sensitized patient can be evidenced by:
    A. hypotension.
    B. bradycardia.
    C. hemataemesis.
    D. hypotonia.

27. An anaphylactic reaction is a function of which body system?
    A. cardiovascular
    B. respiratory
    C. central nervous system
    D. immune

28 Which immunoglobulin is responsible for initiating the anapylactic reaction?
    A. IgE
    B. IgM
    C. IgA
    D. IgD

29. If the body has never been exposed to a specific antigen in an IgE reaction before, the response of the body to the first exposure is:
    A. the same as the expected anaphylactic reaction.
    B. more severe than the expected anaphylactic reaction.
    C. typically does not create an anaphylactic reaction.
    D. creates only a mild anaphylactic reaction.

30. Which of the following would not typically cause an anaphylactic reaction in an individual?
    A. aspirin
    B. x-ray contrast media

C. antacids

D. antibiotics

31. A patient is to receive epinephrine for an allergic reaction. All of the following statements about this administration are true, **except**:

A. 1:1,000 epinephrine should be used for SQ administration.

B. 1:10,000 epinephrine should be used for ET administration.

C. 1:1,000 epinephrine should be used for IV administration.

D. 1:10,000 epinephrine should be used for IV administration.

32. Which of the following clinical symptoms is not a direct result of the chemical mediator release in anaphylaxis?

A. tachycardia

B. dyspnea

C. low blood pressure

D. itching and hives

33. You are conducting an initial assessment of a patient with a history of bee stings to which he is allergic. Which of the following would best indicate that your patient is experiencing a severe reaction?

A. urticaria

B. unresponsiveness

C. bilateral wheezing

D. cool, clammy skin

34. Your initial treatment for a patient with a severe reaction would be:

A. administration of high flow oxygen.

B. c-spine stabilization.

C. initiation of an IV line.

D. administration of epinephrine.

35. Your anaphylactic patient needs endotracheal intubation, and you note severe glottic edema. You should:

A. increase the rate of PPV.

B. perform a needle cricothyrotomy.

C. consider inserting a smaller diameter endotracheal tube.

D. force the tube in between the edematous tissue.

36. Which of the following clinical findings is least suggestive of a severe anaphylactic reaction?

A. extreme anxiety

B. hypotension

C. bilateral wheezing on inspiration and expiration

D. inspiratory stridor

37. In the severe anaphylactic reaction, it is imperative to try and maintain normal perfusion pressures. Which of the following will help with this goal?

A. administration of IV fluids

B. placing a constriction band between the injection site and the heart

C. administration of epinephrine

D. A and C

38. Nausea, vomiting, and diarrhea, when present in an anaphylactic reaction, are all associated with:

A. severe vasodilation.

B. histamine release.

C. bronchoconstriction.

D. none of the above.

39. What type of IV fluid is preferred in the treatment of an anaphylactic patient?

A. isotonic colloid solution

B. hypotonic crystalloid solution

C. hypertonic colloid solution

D. isotonic crystalloid solution

40. After starting an IV in your anaphylactic patient, you decide to administer a fluid bolus because of hypotension. The amount you will infuse is:
    A. 20 ml/kg.
    B. 40 ml/kg.
    C. 10 ml/kg.
    D. 30 ml/kg.

41. Which IV set up will allow the fluid bolus to be administered the fastest?
    A. a 14-gauge with a microdrip administration set
    B. a 20-gauge with a macrodrip administration set
    C. a 16-gauge with a macrodrip administration set
    D. a 18-gauge with a microdrip administration set

42. Which one of the below effects of epinephrine are least desirable when administering it to an anaphylactic shock patient?
    A. beta 1 effects
    B. beta 2 effects
    C. alpha effects
    D. all the above are undesirable in an anaphylactic patient

43. After administering epinephrine to an anaphylactic patient, which of the following findings do you expect to see improvement in?
    A. respiratory distress
    B. low blood pressure
    C. altered mental status
    D. all of the above

44. Which of the epinephrine dosages would be appropriate for a mild allergic reaction?
    A. 0.03 mg
    B. 3.0 mg

C. 0.3 mg
D. none of the above

45. Which of the epinephrine dosages would be appropriate for a severe allergic reaction?
    A. 0.03 mg
    B. 3.0 mg
    C. 0.3 mg
    D. none of the above

46. The major difference between administering epinephrine to a mild and severe allergic reaction is:
    A. the route of administration.
    B. the dose of epinephrine to be administered.
    C. the concentration of epinephrine to be used.
    D. the repeat dose of epinephrine.

47. You have a patient who believes he is having an allergic reaction. The patient has a sudden onset of chest tightness, wheezing, stridor with dyspnea and a poor tidal volume, severe urticaria, erythema, and pruritis. Vitals are B/P 88/palp, HR is 118, and RR is 36. Based upon this presentation, the patient is having:
    A. a severe allergic reaction.
    B. a mild allergic reaction.
    C. a subtle allergic reaction.
    D. no allergic reaction.

48. The mechanism that initiates the most rapid reaction is usually:
    A. ingestion.
    B. inhalation.
    C. injection.
    D. absorption.

49. What is the number-one cause of death in a patient with a severe anaphylactic reaction?
    A. urticaria
    B. glottic edema

C. hypotension

D. bronchoconstriction

50. All of the following treatment options are appropriate for treating a severe anaphylactic patient, **except**:

A. endotracheal intubation.

B. administration of 0.5 mg of epinephrine IV.

C. high flow oxygen.

D. IV therapy of normal saline at a KVO rate.

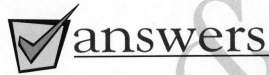

answers & rationales

1.

A. The immune system will, when faced with a foreign substance, create antibodies to eliminate the invading substance. These invading substances known as antigens or allergens, are components of the antigen/antibody reaction seen in acute anaphylactic reactions.

2.

D. Sensitization begins when the body is initially exposed to an antigen. This initiates the production of antibodies specific to that antigen. These antibodies allow the elimination of the antigen on repeated exposures. Chemical mediators are released along with the antibody/antigen reaction. This is what causes the clinical manifestation seen in an allergic reaction.

3.

B. Antibodies are created by plasma cells in response to exposure to an antigen (foreign substance). When manufactured, these antibodies attach themselves to MAST cells and basophils that house the chemical mediators. The other types of cells listed are types of white blood cells useful in fighting infections.

4.

D. Antibodies created by the immune system are designed to eliminate unwanted allergens that may invade the blood stream. This is how the immune system helps to protect the body. Immunoglobulins are also structures created by the immune system to ward off invaders. Basophils are the white blood

cells that the antibodies attach to. Haptens are a type or class of antibodies.

5.

C. An anaphylactic reaction is also characterized as an antigen/antibody reaction. When an antigen (foreign substance) enters the blood stream, antibodies specific to that antigen attack and eliminate it. An acute anaphylactic reaction occurs when there is an overwhelming antigen/antibody reaction.

6.

B. The immune system is responsible for eliminating any foreign substance that gains access to the blood system. In an acute anaphylactic reaction, there is an inappropriate overwhelming response of the immune system. The chemical mediators released in such an emergency create the clinical signs and symptoms seen particularly in the cardiovascular, respiratory, and integumentary systems. It can also involve the gastrointestinal and nervous systems.

7.

B. The laryngeal edema resulting in occlusion of the airway develops rapidly and can be fatal within minutes if untreated. A severe allergic reaction can affect the cardiovascular and respiratory systems with fatal effects. In an acute reaction, the patient can display hypotension, tachycardia, stridor (from laryngeal edema) and bronchoconstriction.

8.

D. Upon introduction of the antigen in an allergic reaction, antibodies cause the release of chemical mediators from MAST cells and basophils which cause changes in the cardiovascular system. These changes include vasodilation, or a decrease in systemic vascular resistance, peripheral pooling of blood, and increased capillary permeability. These changes cause the tachycardia and hypotension seen in acute reactions.

9.

B. Chemical mediators released from MAST cells and basophils in an allergic reaction also affect the pulmonary system by causing profound bronchoconstriction, bronchial wall edema, and increased mucous production. This makes it harder for the person to breathe because of airway occlusion. This is known as an increase in airway resistance.

10.

A. The chemical mediators released in the anaphylactic reaction affect the cardiovascular system significantly. These changes often cause profound hypotension in the acute reaction. Tachycardia occurs as the body attempts to maintain a normal blood pressure by increasing cardiac output. Tachypnea (rapid breathing) may be seen due to hypoxia, but hyperpnea (deep breathing) is not likely due to the respiratory effects seen in anaphylactic reactions.

11.

A. Urticaria (hives) and pruritis (itching) are hallmark signs of an allergic reaction and are caused by the chemical mediators released from MAST cells and basophils. The skin may become reddened (erythemic) from the chemical mediators as well. Cellular changes due to hypoxia or acidosis do not play a role in the development of urticaria or pruritis, but could be associated with cyanosis.

12.

C. Although numerous chemical mediators are released from MAST cells and basophils during an allergic reaction, histamine is one of the most prevalent. Histamine release has cardiovascular, respiratory, and integumentary manifestations. Phos-

phodiasterase is an intracellular enzyme and is not a component of an allergic reaction. Cyclic AMP is a second chemical messenger for cell transmission, and glucagon is a hormone that is involved with blood glucose levels.

13.

D. An acute reaction can occur from any mode of exposure, inhalation, absorption, or ingestion. In essence, if the antigen can gain access to the body, an allergic reaction can occur.

14.

C. Pollen is a common cause of asthmatic attacks and "hay fever" symptoms, however it is not commonly associated with anaphylaxis. Wasp venom from stings, certain medications, and certain foods (nuts, shellfish) are commonly associated with anaphylaxis. Be aware however, that almost any substance could create a reaction.

15.

D. Basophils are a type of white blood cell which is important to the allergic reaction. Since it is a white blood cell, it is found within the blood stream and circulates throughout the body. MAST cells, also important to the allergic reaction, are stationary and are located within the walls of connective tissue, respiratory tree, and vascular smooth muscle.

16.

A. Hallmark integumentary signs seen in anaphylaxis include pruritis and urticaria. Rhinorrhea and erythema may also be present, but are not considered as "hallmark" findings.

17.

C. The anaphylactic patient may present anywhere on the continuum of stable to severe, depending upon their personal reaction to the antigen. However, alterations in the level of consciousness, hypotension, and stridorous respirations are considered as findings in a severe allergic reaction.

18.

B. Bronchoconstriction brought on by chemical mediator release, results in an increase in airway resistance and wheezing. Stridor may be present, but is from laryngeal edema. Crackles are secondary to mucous secretion in larger passages of the airway, not bronchoconstriction. Gurgles are fluid in the alveolar sacs and is not common to allergic reactions.

19.

C. All of the clinical findings listed can be considered significant findings of a severe reaction, however minimal wheezing upon auscultation is most likely indicative of poor air exchange due to bronchoconstriction. This patient is starting to display respiratory failure and cardiac arrest may follow shortly thereafter.

20.

B. Glottic edema from fluid shifting out of the cells due to an increase in capillary permeability creates a narrowing of the glottic opening. As the person inhales against the narrowed opening, it creates stridor. Stridor is a high pitched inspiratory noise indicative of at least 75 percent glottic closure. Wheezing is from bronchoconstriction, while pruritis is the perception of itching. Hemoptysis is coughing up blood.

21.

B. Inspiratory stridor is indicative of greater than 75 percent glottic closure caused by the swelling of the glottic tissues from the anaphylaxis and airway occlusion. This indicates a severe reaction and the patient may require advanced airway interventions. Vasodilation causes a drop in systemic vascular resistance and hypotension.

22.

B. The blood pressure of 86/68, respiratory rate of 42, and heart rate of 130 would be most likely. Vital signs in the severe allergic reaction will be the result of the body's response to the chemical media-

tor release. Generally, the patient will be hypotensive, tachycardic, and tachypneic.

23.

C. Diminishing breath sounds are most likely due to respiratory failure, not improvement. Given the seriousness of the patient initially, and the lack of response to initial treatment the patient's status is most likely deteriorating. With appropriate management, the anaphylactic patient's status should improve in the prehospital environment.

24.

C. The quicker the onset of the anaphylactic reaction, especially after an injection mechanism, the more likely the overall reaction will be more severe.

25.

A. The most severe of reactions can occur within minutes of the exposure, but a severe anaphylactic reaction can occur hours after exposure to the antigen. However, bee stings and intravenous medications, injection mechanisms, are most commonly associated with a rapid onset and serious manifestations.

26.

A. Hypotension from an increase in capillary permeability, a decrease in systemic vascular resistance, and peripheral pooling of blood is the result of histamine release in anaphylaxis. Bradycardia is unlikely since the normal feedback mechanism is tachycardia. Hemataemesis, vomiting blood, is not a common finding and hypotonia is secondary to profound hypoxemia and hypoperfusion and is not directly due to the histamine release.

27.

D. Anaphylaxis is overwhelming response by the immune system to an antigen to which it has been sensitized. It is the immune system that creates the emergency, and its effects are primarily seen in the respiratory, cardiovascular, and central nervous systems.

28.

A. IgE is the one antibody that contributes to allergic and anaphylactic responses. There are five classes of human antibodies, also called immunoglobulins. They include IgM, IgG, IgA, IgE, and IgD. These all play a role in the immune response.

29.

C. The first time an antigen gains access to the body in an IgE-type reaction, there is usually not an anaphylactic reaction until the body becomes sensitized. After the first exposure, the body becomes sensitized (and primed) for an allergic reaction. Typically, subsequent repeated exposures create more severe reactions.

30.

C. Of the listed possibilities, the only one that has not been commonly cited as a probable antigen is antacids. All of the others have been found to create allergic reactions with exposure. Gathering a good history about allergic reactions is very important. Patient needs may make it necessary to alter your protocols.

31.

C. When administering epinephrine for anaphylaxis, there are four things to consider. First, is the reaction severe or mild? This determines the route of administration. Second, what is the desired dose? In either case it is 0.3 to 0.5 mg. Third, what concentration of epi should be used? This depends on route and severity. Basically, IM or SQ epinephrine dilution for a mild reaction is 1:1,000. A severe reaction is 1:10,000 dilution either IVP or ET administration.

32.

A. Tachycardia is a reflex mechanism for hypoxia and hypotension that accompanies anaphylaxis and is a common manifestation of a mild or severe reaction. Dyspnea is caused by the bronchoconstriction and airway edema, and low blood pressure is a result of severe peripheral vasodilation and increased capillary permeability. The itching and hives are from histamine release and capillary dilation.

33.

B. During the initial assessment, you are looking for significantly life-threatening conditions to the airway, breathing, and circulation. If you are assessing a patient thought to be having an anaphylactic reaction and they present as unresponsive, this is a grave sign of severe hypoxemia and cerebral hypoperfusion. The other findings may well be present, but may also be seen with a milder reaction.

34.

A. During the primary assessment you treat life-threats as they are discovered. Someone unresponsive due to anaphylaxis needs oxygen above all else first. After the oxygenation, you would initiate an IV and give epinephrine according to need. Immobilization is only necessary if you suspect some type of traumatic incident.

35.

C. If possible, try using a smaller diameter tube that may fit in the edematous glottic opening. Any airway is better than none as PPV will be totally ineffective if the glottic opening completely swells shut. Forcing a tube through is damaging. Performing a needle cricothyrotomy is beyond the scope of an EMT-I.

36.

A. Extreme anxiety may be present in a patient who has been exposed to an antigen to which they know they are allergic. The person may be aware that they can have a severe reaction and may be scared. Additionally, the release of catecholamines early in the anaphylactic process may precipitate anxiety. The other findings are more suggestive of a moderate to severe reaction.

37.

D. Administration of intravenous fluids will increase intravascular volume which might raise perfusion pressures. The concentration of epinephrine will cause vasoconstriction and increase perfusion pressure by raising SVR.

38.

B. Histamine release can cause the patient to experience nausea, vomiting, and diarrhea. This effect is enhanced by the increased capillary permeability as more fluid enters the intestinal tract. Vasodilation and bronchoconstriction occur as a result of histamine as well, but they do not cause the GI distress.

39.

D. Fluids such as normal saline and lactated Ringer's are isotonic crystalloid solutions that will immediately increase intravascular volume in the anaphylactic patient. Hypotonic and hypertonic solutions are generally not available to prehospital providers.

40.

A. Whenever you have a fluid depleted patient the standard bolus amount is 20 ml/kg infused at a wide-open rate. Following this, reassess your patient to see if you need to repeat the bolus.

41.

C. When infusing a large amount of fluid in a short amount of time, use a set-up that utilizes a large-bore angiocatheter (14 or 16 gauge), and a macro-drip administration set. Also if possible, use the shortest catheter possible, like an inch and a quarter. These steps will reduce the resistance to flow as much as possible.

42.

A. Beta 1 stimulation is the least desirable in an anaphylactic reaction. This causes an increase in cardiac activity that will then require more perfusion and oxygenation. Beta 2 causes smooth muscle relaxation of the bronchioles and alpha causes peripheral vasoconstriction.

43.

D. Because of the effects of epinephrine administration, you can expect to see all the above findings. Respiratory distress should diminish due to beta 2 stimulation, the blood pressure should normalize from vasoconstriction and the orientation should improve with enhanced oxygenation and perfusion to the CNS.

44.

C. Epinephrine for a mild allergic reaction is 0.3 to 0.5 milligrams of a 1:1,000 solution administered SQ or IM.

45.

C. Epinephrine for a severe allergic reaction is 0.3 to 0.5 milligrams of a 1:10,000 solution administered IV push or via the ET tube.

46.

A. The most significant difference is the route of administration. The route of administration will determine the concentration. For SQ or IM, 1:1,000 is used. For a severe reaction you use 1:10,000 IV or ET. The dose remains the same regardless of the route or severity of the reaction.

47.

A. These clinical findings are most consistent with a severe allergic reaction. The major clinical findings that demonstrate a severe reaction are hypotension, stridor, severe wheezing, and an altered mental status. The skin findings are also found with a mild reaction but persist through a severe reaction.

48.

C. Given the rapid onset, the most probable cause is an injection mechanism. This places the antigen within the body where it may be immediately absorbed and transported.

49.

B. The number one-cause of death in any severe ana-phylactic reaction is glottic edema causing an airway obstruction. That is why airway maintenance is so important, and the presence of inspiratory stridor a significant finding. Severe bronchoconstriction and hypotension can also be fatal, but its presentation is not as rapid as the glottic edema.

50.

D. The IV at a KVO rate is inappropriate. The IV should be a 20 ml/kg bolus run at a wide-open rate. Treatment of a severe allergic reaction must occur rapidly if the patient is to have a successful recovery. The cornerstones of treatment are reversal of the bronchoconstriction, oxygenation, correcting vasodilation, and restoring intravascular volume.

11 Pharmacology

chapter objectives

The questions in this chapter serve as a supplement to the curriculum and have no direct relation to the DOT objectives.

DIRECTIONS Each of the questions or incomplete statements below is followed by suggested answers or completions. Select the **one answer** that is best in each case.

1. After administering a nitroglycerin tablet sublingually, a patient complains of a bitter, burning sensation under his tongue. Your next course of action would be to:
   A. explain to the patient that this is normal.
   B. instruct the patient to immediately chew and swallow the tablet.
   C. give the patient approximately 8 oz of water.
   D. instruct the patient to immediately spit the tablet out.

2. You are examining a 45-year-old male who complains of substernal chest pain. The patient states that after onset, he took 2 unprescribed nitroglycerin tablets he found in a friend's medicine cabinet. What action would be appropriate in reference to the nitroglycerin?
   A. examine the nitroglycerin and container.
   B. instruct the patient to swallow a third tablet from the container.
   C. contact the physician whose name is on the container.
   D. instruct the patient to take another nitroglycerin tablet from the container.

3. Select the proper route and dosage for a single administration of nitroglycerin.
   A. sublingual spray at 4 mg/spray
   B. sublingual tablet at 0.4 mg/tablet
   C. sublingual spray at 4 g/spray
   D. sublingual tablet at 1/100 gr/tablet

4. Which of the following is the most appropriate order of treatment for a patient with chest pain who has never taken nitroglycerin before?
   A. nitroglycerin, IV
   B. IV, nitroglycerin, oxygen
   C. IV, nitroglycerin
   D. oxygen, IV, nitroglycerin

5. You are assessing a patient involved in a motor vehicle accident. The patient suffered blunt trauma to the chest and abdomen and is complaining of substernal chest pain that radiates to the left shoulder. The patient is anxious and presents with vital signs of: BP 108/58, HR 136, RR 32, and skin that is cool and diaphoretic. Appropriate management of this patient would include:
   A. oxygen, full immobilization, IV, nitroglycerin.
   B. oxygen, IV, transport.
   C. oxygen, full immobilization, IV.
   D. oxygen, full immobilization, nitroglycerin, IV.

6. In which of the following would the administration of nitroglycerin be beneficial?
   A. shock
   B. seizures
   C. congestive heart failure
   D. allergic reactions

7. Which of the following represents a possible adverse reaction to nitroglycerin?
   A. bronchial constriction
   B. hypertension
   C. tachycardia
   D. pupillary constriction

8. Which of the following best describes the mechanism by which nitroglycerin reduces chest pain?

   A. decreasing cardiac workload
   B. increase in cardiac contractility
   C. constriction of the coronary arteries
   D. dilation of the bronchioles

9. Which of the following best describes why a nitroglycerin tablet is administered sublingually?

   A. to avoid gastric irritation
   B. to discourage possible vomiting
   C. to avoid aspiration of the tablet
   D. to promote rapid absorption

10. You are assessing a 60-year-old male whose chief complaint is substernal chest pain accompanied by shortness of breath and diaphoresis. The patient has a history of cardiac problems and presents with vital signs of: BP 86/72, HR 68, RR 24. Appropriate management of this individual would consist of:

    A. oxygen, IV of normal saline
    B. oxygen, IV, nitroglycerin 0.4 mg
    C. oxygen, IV, nitroglycerin 0.2 mg
    D. oxygen, nitroglycerin 4 mg

11. Which of the following best describes the action of diazepam in seizure control?

    A. It inhibits seizure activity by depressing the medulla.
    B. It suppresses the spread of seizure activity through the motor cortex.
    C. It prevents seizures by activating the parasympathetic nervous system.
    D. It is a potent central nervous system stimulant which prevents the formation of seizures.

12. To manage an adult patient in status epilepticus, the dosage of diazepam is:

    A. 1–5 mg IV.
    B. 5–10 mg IV.
    C. 10–15 mg IV.
    D. 15–20 mg IV.

13. Identify the correct drug class for diazepam.

    A. anti-depressants
    B. depressants
    C. narcotics
    D. benzodiazepine

14. When administering diazepam intravenously, it should be given slowly to:

    A. minimize venous irritation.
    B. speed up the action of the drug.
    C. avoid hypersensitivity reactions.
    D. prevent accidental overdose.

15. Diazepam would be indicated in all of the following situations, **except**:

    A. acute anxiety states.
    B. status epilepticus.
    C. unconsciousness of unknown origin.
    D. major motor seizures.

16. After administering diazepam to your patient, you observe that he is drowsy and that his blood pressure and respiratory rate have slightly decreased. You know that this occurred because:

    A. he is hypersensitive to the medication.
    B. he received an accidental overdose.
    C. these are common side effects of this drug.
    D. you administered the medication too slowly.

17. Your pediatric patient is in status epilepticus. What is the correct dosage of diazepam in this situation?

    A. 0.1–0.3 mg/kg
    B. 0.5–2 mg/kg
    C. 2–5 mg
    D. 5–10 mg

18. Diazepam should not be mixed with other drugs because it may cause:
   A. a severe hypersensitivity reaction.
   B. an accidental overdose.
   C. precipitation within the IV line or vein.
   D. drowsiness.

19. The preferred route for the emergency administration of diazepam is:
   A. oral.
   B. sublingual.
   C. intramuscular.
   D. intravenous.

20. Diazepam is used as a premedication for cardioversion primarily because it:
   A. calms the patient and depresses the central nervous system.
   B. reduces anxiety and diminishes the patient's recall.
   C. relaxes skeletal muscles and prevents pain after the procedure.
   D. is relatively short-acting and does not cause hypersensitivity.

21. Which of the following most accurately describes the effect of 50% Dextrose?
   A. causes a decrease in the patient's blood pressure
   B. raises the blood glucose level
   C. promotes bronchodilation
   D. causes peripheral vasoconstriction

22. 50% Dextrose is administered to manage:
   A. hypoglycemia.
   B. seizures.
   C. head injury.
   D. hypertension.

23. A major contraindication to the administration of 50% Dextrose is:

A. acute renal failure.
B. acute stroke.
C. seizures.
D. tachycardia.

24. The proper dose of 50% Dextrose in the adult patient is:
   A. 20 mg
   B. 25 g
   C. 1 mg/kg
   D. none of the above

25. What is the major risk associated with the administration of 50% Dextrose:
   A. tachycardia.
   B. respiratory hypoventilation.
   C. tissue necrosis with extravation.
   D. lowered blood pressure.

26. Thiamine is known more commonly as a:
   A. drug for headaches.
   B. muscle relaxer.
   C. vitamin.
   D. hormone.

27. The mechanism of action for thiamine is to:
   A. increase the transfer of glucose into cells.
   B. allow sugar to last longer for cellular metabolism.
   C. increase sugar absorption from the small intestine.
   D. increase the energy gained from the metabolism of sugar.

28. Thiamine can be administered by:
   A. IV push and IM.
   B. SQ injection.
   C. IM injection and rectally.
   D. IV only.

29. The appropriate dose of thiamine in the pre-hospital environment is:
    A. 100 mg.
    B. 1 mg/kg.
    C. 10 grams.
    D. none of the above.

30. What is the major contraindication associated with the administration of thiamine?
    A. hypoglycemia
    B. hypotension
    C. hypovolemia
    D. hypersensitivity

31. Which of the following best describes the mechanism of action of epinephrine?
    A. stimulates the sympathetic nervous system
    B. stimulates the parasympathetic nervous system
    C. blocks the central nervous system
    D. reduces peripheral vascular resistance

32. The property that makes epinephrine most desirable in cardiac arrest is:
    A. beta 1 stimulation.
    B. beta 2 stimulation.
    C. alpha stimulation.
    D. dopaminergic stimulation.

33. What is the preferred concentration and route for epinephrine in cardiac arrest?
    A. 1:1,000 concentration via IM or SQ administration
    B. 1:10,000 concentration via IVP or endotracheally
    C. 1:1,000 concentration via IVP or endotracheally
    D. 1:10,000 concentration via IM or SQ

34. What is the initial dose for epinephrine in cardiac arrest?
    A. 10 mcg
    B. 1 mcg
    C. 1 mg
    D. 10 mg

35. All of the following are potential side effects of epinephrine, **except**:
    A. palpitations.
    B. bradycardia.
    C. hypertension.
    D. pallor.

36. Which of the following drugs can adsorb poisons that have been ingested?
    A. ipecac
    B. procardia
    C. activated charcoal
    D. oral glucose

37. The dose of activated charcoal for an adult patient is:
    A. 50 g.
    B. 50 mg.
    C. 5 oz.
    D. 1 mg/kg.

38. An indication for the administration of Benadryl is:
    A. anaphylaxis.
    B. coma of unknown origin.
    C. nausea and vomiting.
    D. asthma attacks.

39. The usual adult dose of Benadryl is:
    A. 5 mg/kg.
    B. 50 mg/kg.
    C. 50 milligrams.
    D. 5 grams.

40. The mechanism of action for Benadryl is to:
    A. block histamine release.
    B. block histamine receptors.
    C. block beta receptor sites.
    D. block alpha receptor sites.

41. Which of the following is **not** a beta 2 specific drug that can be administered by a nebulizer?
    A. Ventolin
    B. Bronkosol
    C. Alupent
    D. Somophyllin

42. A beta 2 drug is considered a:
    A. sympathetic agonist.
    B. parasympathetic agonist.
    C. sympathetic antagonist.
    D. parasympathetic antagonist.

43. What is the primary action of a beta 2 drug?
    A. vasodilation
    B. increased heart rate
    C. brochodilation
    D. positive inotropy

44. The proper dose for Albuterol is:
    A. 3.0 mg in 3 ml of normal saline.
    B. 2.5 mg in 2.5 ml of normal saline.
    C. 1.0 mg in 5 ml of normal saline.
    D. 0.5 mg in 2.5 ml of normal saline.

45. The primary indication for the use of a beta 2 specific drug is:
    A. congestive heart failure.
    B. pneumonia.
    C. bronchoconstriction.
    D. myocardial infarction.

46. Which of the following drugs would be used in the management of the hypoglycemic patient?
    A. Albuterol
    B. glycogen
    C. glucagon
    D. Inderal

47. Which of the following would be an indication for the use of glucagon?
    A. patient who overdosed on propranolol
    B. patient with an altered mental status and a blood glucose level of 240 mg/dl
    C. patient with an altered mental status from ingestion of diazepam
    D. liver failure associated with acetominophen overdose

48. Glucagon can best be described as a(n):
    A. drug made up of glucose.
    B. hormone secreted by the alpha cells in the pancreas.
    C. antiarrythmic agent to control PVCs.
    D. drug used to reverse thiamine deficiency.

49. Which of the following best describes the mechanism of action of glucagon?
    A. The glucose contained within the drug raises the blood glucose level.
    B. It decreases the inotropic and chronotropic properties of the heart.
    C. It stimulates an increase in insulin production and secretion allowing the glucose to enter the cells.
    D. It stimulates the liver to convert glycogen stores into free glucose.

50. You are managing a hypoglycemic patient and are unable to establish an IV. What would be the correct dose for glucagon?
    A. 0.25 mg
    B. 0.5 mg
    C. 1.0 mg
    D. 2.5 mg

51. Naloxone is classified as a:
    A. narcotic agonist.
    B. central nervous system stimulant.
    C. narcotic antagonist.
    D. benzodiazepine antagonist.

52. On which of the following drugs would Narcan have no effect?
    A. Demerol
    B. Fentanyl
    C. Nubain
    D. Valium

53. When administering Narcan, which of the following criteria could be used to determine when the appropriate dose has been reached?
    A. The patient becomes alert and combative.
    B. The respiratory depression has been reversed.
    C. The patient's blood increases by 10 mmHg.
    D. The pupils dilate from a constricted state.

54. What would be considered a contraindication for use of Narcan?
    A. a patient who has had a bad reaction to it before
    B. if the patient has ingested alcohol with the narcotic agent
    C. if the drug ingested or injected is a synthetic narcotic
    D. if the patient is comatose from the drug overdose

55. From your history, you gather that the unresponsive patient has ingested a large number of Darvon pills and drank a fifth of whiskey. The proper dose of Narcan in this case would be:
    A. 1 mg IV.
    B. 2 mg ET.
    C. 5 mg IV.
    D. 25 mg ET.

56. Which of the following is a first-line drug in the treatment of ventricular dysrhythmias?
    A. magnesium sulfate
    B. atropine
    C. lidocaine
    D. bretylium

57. Which of the following is **not** an indication for the administration of lidocaine?
    A. multifocal PVCs
    B. salvos of PVCs
    C. couplets
    D. P on R phenomenon

58. You have administered a bolus of lidocaine to a patient experiencing PVCs. The PVCs are abolished after the bolus. Your next action should be to:
    A. start an infusion of lidocaine at 2 mg/minute.
    B. administer a second bolus at 1.5 mg/kg.
    C. monitor the patient and rebolus with lidocaine at 0.5 mg/kg if any ectopy occurs.
    D. increase the oxygen and continue to monitor the patient.

59. Which of the following is a contraindication to the use of lidocaine?
    A. pulseless ventricular tachycardia
    B. refractory ventricular fibrillation over 20 minutes in duration
    C. PVCs occurring in symptomatic bradycardia
    D. a patient with a history of liver disease

60. The initial dose of lidocaine in a pulseless patient with ventricular tachycardia is:
    A. 0.5 mg/kg.
    B. 1.0 to 1.5 mg/kg.
    C. 2 mg/minute.
    D. 3.0 mg/kg.

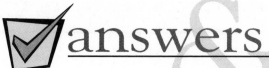

1.

A. A burning or stinging sensation the patient may experience when taking nitroglycerin is considered normal and often indicates the potency of the tablet or spray. In this situation, the EMT-Intermediate should explain to the patient that this is a normal side effect with the medication and will pass in a few minutes.

2.

A. The EMT-Intermediate must examine the nitroglycerin and container. More specifically, the condition and expiration date must be determined. Nitroglycerin tends to deteriorate rapidly after exposure to air and light and lose its efficacy after the medicine has expired. This may explain the failure of the nitroglycerin to alleviate this individual's chest pain. Instructing the patient to take another pill from the same container is inappropriate in that this medication has been prescribed for someone else. Contacting the physician whose name is on the container will do little for the patient.

3.

B. Nitroglycerin can be administered by either sublingual tablet or sublingual spray. The correct dosage for a single dose would be 0.4 mg or 1/150 grain.

4.

D. The correct order of intervention is best represented by: oxygen, IV, nitroglycerin. Oxygen is always a first-line drug in the management of chest pain. An IV should be established prior to the administration of the nitroglycerin for the patient who has never received the drug before, just in case the patient has an adverse reaction to the medication and requires immediate fluids and/or other medications.

5.

C. The most appropriate care for this patient is oxygen, full immobilization, IV en route, and no nitroglycerin. This patient appears to be in compensatory shock as indicated by the mechanism of injury and vital signs. Nitroglycerin and its vasodilation effect are contraindicated in the presence of shock. Also, there is no true indication for administration of nitroglycerin.

6.

C. Nitroglycerin may be beneficial to the patient suffering the effects of congestive heart failure. The nitroglycerin causes vasodilation, which can decrease the quantity of blood returning to the heart, and a decrease in peripheral vascular resistance. In congestive heart failure, there is more blood entering the heart than the heart can effectively pump. This results in pulmonary edema, associated respiratory distress, and hypoxia.

7.

C. Tachycardia may be a side effect of nitroglycerin. The vasodilatory aspects of nitroglycerin reduce the blood return to the myocardium and this results in a corresponding reduction in the cardiac output. Blood pressure is often decreased and if it is lowered to the point of significant hypotension, the body will attempt to compensate with an increase in the heart rate. This is in an attempt to deliver more oxygenated blood to the cells. This is the reason that many authorities state that the systolic blood pressure should be lowered only 10 percent of its initial value. Bronchial constriction, hypertension, and pupillary constriction are not physiological side effects to the administration of nitroglycerin.

8.

A. Nitroglycerin is a smooth muscle relaxant that reduces cardiac workload. During times of stress or exercise the heart often needs more oxygen than narrowed coronary arteries can supply. Relaxing the peripheral arteries reduces resistance and, to some extent, dilating the coronary arteries increases coronary blood flow and perfusion to the ischemic cells.

9.

D. Because the underside of the tongue is rich in capillaries, sublingual administration of nitroglycerin tablets promotes rapid absorption and therefore fast drug action in the body.

10.

A. Appropriate management of this patient would include oxygen and a crystalloid IV. Nitroglycerin is contraindicated in this situation due to a state of hypotension.

11.

B. Diazepam is an effective agent to control seizure activity because it suppresses the spread of seizure activity through the motor cortex of the brain.

12.

B. To manage status epilepticus, the dosage of diazepam is 5 to 10 mg IV, titrated to effect.

13.

D. Diazepam is in the drug class known as benzodiazepines.

14.

A. When administering diazepam intravenously, it should be given slowly to minimize venous irritation and hypotension.

15.

C. It would be inappropriate to give diazepam to manage an unconsciousness of unknown origin or one who is known to be hypersensitive. Diazepam is indicated for the management of acute anxiety states, status epilepticus, and major motor seizures.

16.

C. After administering diazepam, it is not unusual to observe drowsiness or decreases in your patient's blood pressure or respiratory rate. These are common side effects of this medication.

17.

A. The correct dosage of diazepam for the management of pediatric status epilepticus is 0.1 to 0.3 mg/kg. Pediatric doses are always based on weight.

18.

C. Diazepam should not be mixed with other drugs because it may cause possible precipitation in the IV line or in the vein.

19.

D. The intravenous route is preferred for the emergency administration of diazepam. An alternative route of administration for pediatric patients is rectal.

20.

B. Diazepam is an effective premedication for cardioversion and other procedures because it reduces anxiety and diminishes the patient's recall.

21.

B. 50% Dextrose is a drug that is sugar in a form that the body can immediately utilize. It should be used in situations where the patient presents with signs and symptoms of hypoglycemia.

22.

A. Since dextrose effectively raises the blood sugar level, it should be administered to those persons that have an altered mental status with a BGL level of (generally) less than 50 mg/dl. It can be used for unresponsiveness, but only if it is assumed to be hypoglycemia related.

23.

B. The major contraindication of the administration of 50% Dextrose is in a patient with increased intracranial pressure from a stroke or head trauma. In these persons, dextrose has been shown to increase intracranial pressure and worsen neurological outcomes. Only administer it to stroke or head-injured patients if hypoglycemia is confirmed.

24.

B. The correct dose for 50% Dextrose in the hypoglycemic patient is 25 g. This usually comes packaged as 25 g in 50 ml of solution and is labeled as 50% Dextrose in water.

25.

C. 50% Dextrose is very hypertonic, and if it is administered in anything less than a patent IV line extravation can occur. When this happens tissue necrosis is often the result.

26.

C. Thiamine is known more commonly as vitamin B_1. It is necessary for the full mobilization of energy from sugar sources. It is not manufactured by the body so thiamine must come from the diet.

27.

D. Thiamine is a vitamin that is not made by the body, but is necessary for the conversion of pyruvic acid into acetyl-coenzyme-A. Without this step, a large majority of energy available in glucose cannot be used.

28.

D. The preferred route for thiamine administration is IV push. However, in the absence of an IV line, it can be administered deep IM.

29.

A. The dose for thiamine is 100 mg. It is the same dose regardless if it is administered IV push or intramuscularly.

30.

D. In the emergency setting, there are no contraindications to the use of this drug with the exception of known hypersensitivity to the drug.

31.

A. Epinephrine is a drug that stimulates adrenergic receptors. That classifies this drug as a sympathomimetic, one that stimulates the sympathetic nervous system.

32.

C. Epinephrine stimulates alpha and beta sites equally. In cardiac arrest however, it is the alpha effects that are most desirable. These alpha effects cause an increase in vasoconstriction which will increase perfusion pressures generated during the administration of external chest compressions.

33.

B. Epinephrine in cardiac arrest should be administered via IV push or down the endotracheal tube. Either of these routes will allow immediate absorption and improved circulation in the body. When given IV push, 1 mg of 1:10,000 solution should be used. When given down the ET tube the dose is increased 2 to 2.5 times.

34.

C. The initial IV push dose of epinephrine in cardiac arrest is 1 milligram. It can be repeated every 3 to 5 minutes at the same dose or increased to 3 mg, 5 mg, or 0.1 mg/Kg.

35.

B. Since epinephrine is a drug that stimulates the sympathetic nervous system the side effects will include palpitations, possible hypertension, nausea/vomiting, and tachycardia and pale skin.

36.

C. Activated charcoal is a drug that, when administered soon after an ingestion poisoning, adsorbs (binds) the poison so that it can pass through the gastrointestinal tract in a whole form without being absorbed. The porous charcoal minimizes absorption into the body. Ipecac is an emetic agent, procardia is a calcium channel blocker, and oral glucose is for hypoglycemic emergencies.

37.

A. The correct adult dose is 50 to 75 grams.

38.

A. Benadryl (diphenhydramine) is an antihistamine used to counteract the effects of histamine release. It is used in those instances when there is a large amount of histamine release within the body, such as anaphylaxis or allergic reactions. It is not warranted in a coma of unknown etiology and is contraindicated for asthma.

39.

C. The adult dose of Benadryl is 25 to 50 mg IV push or IM. Of the two routes, the IV administration is preferred.

40.

B. The major mechanism of action for Benadryl is the blockage of histamine receptor sites thereby blocking histamine action. It cannot influence the amount of histamine released in response to the antigen.

41.

D. Somophyllin has beta 2 properties, however it cannot be delivered by nebulizer. This drug is usually administered as an IV infusion.

42.

A. A beta 2 drug is considered a sympathetic agonist because it has beta 2 properties that mimic those of the sympathetic nervous system resulting in bronchodilation. An antagonist has properties that act against the sympathetic nervous system. Even though a parasympathetic antagonist, like Atropine, would reverse bronchoconstriction, it does not contain beta 2 properties.

43.

C. The primary action of a beta 2 drug is bronchodilation. Some vascular smooth muscle dilation will also result from beta 2 stimulation. An increased heart rate (chronotropic effect) and increased contractility of the myocardium (inotropic effect) occur from beta 1 properties.

44.

B. The proper dose of Albuterol is 2.5 mg mixed in 2.5 ml of normal saline for nebulization. The total amount mixed is 0.5 ml of a 0.5% solution.

45.

C. The primary indication for the use of a beta 2 specific drug is bronchoconstriction associated with bronchial asthma, emphysema, chronic bronchitis, and COPD.

46.

C. Glucagon is an alternative drug that can be used in the treatment of a patient who is hypoglycemic. It is a hormone that stimulates the conversion of liver glycogen to glucose, thereby raising the blood glucose level. It is only effective if glycogen stores are available. Intravenous 50% Dextrose remains the number one drug of choice in the management of hypoglycemia.

47.

A. Glucagon is also used in the treatment of beta blocker overdose. Propranolol is a beta blocker.

48.

B. Glucagon is a protein hormone that is secreted by the alpha cells in the pancreas. It does not contain any glucose.

49.

D. Glucagon raises the blood glucose level by stimulating the conversion of glycogen, the stored form of glucose in the liver, back into free glucose that enters the blood and is available for use by the cells. This in turn raises the blood glucose level.

50.

C. The typical dose is 1.0 mg. Glucagon is normally administered as an IM injection in the hypoglycemic patient. If an IV was established, 50% Dextrose should be administered and not glucagon.

51.

C. Naloxone is considered a narcotic antagonist. It competes for opiate binding sites or blocks the ability of the opiate or narcotic to bind at a receptor site.

52.

D. Narcan will not reverse the effects of benzodiazepines, like valium. Demerol, Fentanyl, and Nubain are all narcotic substances. Narcan only will affect and block opiate derivatives or synthetic narcotics.

53.

B. As a general rule, the appropriate dose of narcan is enough to reverse any respiratory depression or hypotension associated with the narcotic. It is not recommended that enough be given to completely arouse the patient because most patients become agitated and violent when completely responsive.

54.

A. The only contraindication to the use of narcan is hypersensitivity to the drug.

55.

C. Darvon typically requires larger doses of Narcan to achieve a response. In this case, 5 mg of Narcan would be an appropriate dose to use to try to elicit a response from the patient.

56.

C. Lidocaine is the drug of choice in the treatment of most ventricular dysrhythmias. Bretylium is often the second line drug to be used. Atropine is used to treat bradydysrhythmias. Magnesium sulfate is a third line drug of choice in the treatment of ventricular fibrillation and first line in torsades de pointes.

57.

D. P on R phenomenon is not an indictation. However, R on T, where the R wave of the QRS complex is falling on or near the T wave is an indication for administration of lidocaine. The R on T phenomenon can easily precipitate ventricular fibrillation or ventricular tachycardia.

58.

A. Once you have abolished the ectopy using a lidocaine bolus, it is necessary to maintain the therapeutic dose by starting an infusion. The infusion ranges from 2 mg/minute to 4 mg/minute. In this case, since only one dose of 1.0 mg/kg was administered, an infusion set at 2 mg/minute is used.

59.

C. PVCs occurring in bradycardia are typically to compensate for the low heart rate. The treatment of choice is atropine or pacing to increase the heart rate and hopefully abolish the PVCs. If the heart rate is increased above 60/minute and the PVCs continue, consider the administration of lidocaine.

60.

B. Pulseless ventricular tachycardia is managed the same as ventricular fibrillation. The initial dose of lidocaine is 1.0 to 1.5 mg/kg IV bolus.

12 Anatomy and Physiology

chapter objectives

The questions in this chapter serve as a supplement to the curriculum and have no direct relation to the DOT objectives.

DIRECTIONS Each of the questions or incomplete statements below is followed by suggested answers or completions. Select the **one answer** that is best in each case.

1. Which of the following best illustrates a major function of smooth muscle?
   A. formation of the heart
   B. maintenance of blood pressure
   C. connect bone to bone
   D. move the skeleton

2. You are assessing a patient who has been slashed with a knife on the back of the hand over the middle of the metacarpals. The wound is very deep and the patient complains of great difficulty in moving his index and middle fingers. Which of the following structures do you suspect to be damaged?
   A. tendons
   B. ligaments
   C. cartilage
   D. ulna and radius

3. Skeletal muscles promote the primary movement of the human body through which of the following actions?
   A. relaxation
   B. voluntary stretching
   C. involuntary stretching
   D. contraction

4. Which of the following illustrates a prime function of the muscular system?
   A. provides the body with structure
   B. prevents internal fluid loss
   C. moves the skeletal bones
   D. provides for the storage of fat

5. You are assessing a 23-year-old male who states that he twisted his left knee while playing football. Assessment reveals ecchymosis and edema in the area of the injury. Which of the following choices best represents the most appropriate management of this injury?
   A. application of a pressure bandage
   B. immobilization of the extremity
   C. application of ice only
   D. transport in a position of comfort

6. Within the human body, the kidneys function to:
   A. form feces.
   B. cleanse blood plasma of waste.
   C. regulate body temperature.
   D. absorb glucose from the blood.

7. A patient has been struck in the back with a baseball bat. Upon assessment, you note an obvious fracture to the twelfth rib along the midscapular line on the left side. Which of the following organs would you suspect may possibly be injured?
   A. bladder
   B. stomach
   C. liver
   D. kidney

8. Urine moves through the urinary system in which order?
   A. ureter, kidney, urethra, bladder
   B. kidney, urethra, bladder, ureter
   C. kidney, ureter, bladder, urethra
   D. urethra, kidney, bladder, ureter

9. Which of the following choices best de-scribes location of the urinary bladder?
   A. pelvic cavity, posterior to the pubic bone
   B. abdominal cavity, adjacent to the gallbladder
   C. pelvic cavity, posterior to the vertebrae
   D. abdominal cavity, directly behind the umbilicus

10. Which of the following would the EMT-Intermediate be most likely to observe in acute renal failure?
    A. vomiting of blood
    B. decreased urinary output
    C. blood in the stool
    D. increased urinary output

11. The production of sperm and secretion of hormones is the function of the:
    A. penis.
    B. scrotum.
    C. testes.
    D. vas deferens.

12. The primary male sex hormone is:
    A. gonadtropin.
    B. testosterone.
    C. estrogen.
    D. luteinizing hormone.

13. The female reproductive system is comprised of the ovaries, uterus, and:
    A. vagina.
    B. estrogen.
    C. ova.
    D. bladder.

14. The primary female sex hormone is:
    A. estrogen.
    B. testosterone.
    C. gonadtropin.
    D. luteinizing hormone.

15. Which organ is responsible for the exchange of oxygen and nutrients between maternal and fetal circulation:
    A. endometrium.
    B. vagina.
    C. uterus.
    D. placenta.

16. The endocrine organ known as the "master gland" is the:
    A. pancreas.
    B. pituitary.
    C. thymus.
    D. thyroid.

17. The hormone which enhances uterine con-traction and stimulates milk production in the mammary glands is:
    A. follicle stimulating hormone.
    B. human growth hormone.
    C. vasopressin.
    D. oxytocin.

18. Hormones produced by the medulla of the adrenal glands:
    A. increase blood pressure by increasing heart rate and strength of contraction, and constricting peripheral blood vessels.
    B. maintain blood pressure and force of con-traction by slowing heart rate and dilating peripheral blood vessels.
    C. produce bronchoconstriction, increase the rate of digestion, decrease blood glucose levels, and inhibit metabolism.
    D. produce pupillary constriction, increase the rate of digestion, slow heart rate, and dilate peripheral blood vessels.

19. Which of the following pairs of hormones se-creted by the pancreas work in opposition to each other?
    A. glucagon and somatostatin
    B. pancreatic polypeptide and insulin

C. glucagon and insulin

D. insulin and somatostatin

20. Diabetes mellitus is a common metabolic disorder which occurs as a result of:
   A. excessive production of insulin.
   B. excessive production of glucagon.
   C. inadequate production of insulin.
   D. inadequate production of glucagon.

21. The chamber of the heart that receives de-oxygenated blood from the body is the:
   A. left atrium.
   B. right ventricle.
   C. left ventricle.
   D. right atrium.

22. The chordae tendonae are located:
   A. on the ventricular side of the AV valves.
   B. on the ventricular side of the aortic and pulmonic valve.
   C. outside the epicardium, supporting the heart in the pericardial sac.
   D. on the atrial side of the mitral valve.

23. Which of the following is **not** a property of myocardial cells?
   A. conductivity
   B. reactivity
   C. automaticity
   D. contractility

24. Which of the following statements best represents blood flow through the heart?
   A. left atrium, left ventricle, lungs, right atrium, right ventricle
   B. right atrium, right ventricle, lungs, left atrium, left ventricle
   C. right atrium, left atrium, lungs, left ventricle

D. right atrium, right ventricle, lungs, left ventricle, aorta

25. A significant increase in the heart rate above 160 beats/minute will potentially:
   A. decrease cardiac output.
   B. lower oxygen requirements of the heart.
   C. increase stroke volume.
   D. result in increased coronary artery perfusion.

26. If a patient receives a medication to increase the force of myocardial contraction, this will primarily affect:
   A. heart rate.
   B. stroke volume.
   C. peripheral vascular resistance.
   D. none of the above.

27. The primary pacemaker of the heart is the:
   A. sinoatrial node.
   B. intraatrial pathways.
   C. atrioventricular node.
   D. bundle of His.

28. Which of the following usually has no effect on heart rate?
   A. increased sympathetic tone
   B. increased parasympathetic tone
   C. lowered dopaminergic tone
   D. enhanced vagal tone

29. If a drug increases the force of ventricular contraction, it would be termed as a positive _____ agent.
   A. chronotropic
   B. dromotropic
   C. inotropic
   D. isotropic

30. Which of the following heart valves would be responsible for causing pulmonary edema if it allows regurgitation of blood?
    A. tricuspid
    B. pulmonic
    C. bicuspid
    D. aortic

31. Which one of the following organs should **not** be categorized as part of the gastrointestinal system?
    A. pancreas
    B. stomach
    C. rectum
    D. adrenal glands

32. The purpose of the pancreas is to:
    A. act as both an exocrine and endocrine gland.
    B. release stored glycogen back in to the bloodstream.
    C. produce bile for the small intestine.
    D. release estrogen into the blood stream.

33. After clearing the stomach, food passes into the:
    A. jejunum.
    B. duodenum.
    C. ileum.
    D. ascending colon.

34. Food is propelled along the course of the small and large intestines by the rhythmic contraction waves known as:
    A. peristalsis.
    B. paresis.
    C. portal waves.
    D. muscular intropy.

35. The role of the gallbladder is to:
    A. produce bile.
    B. house urine until it is removed by the body.

C. store bile until needed.
    D. none of the above

36. When the protective mucosal lining of the stomach is lost, the acids of the stomach start to erode the stomach wall. This is called:
    A. gastritis.
    B. gastric ulcers.
    C. diverticulitis.
    D. appendicitis.

37. If a perforation were to occur in the proximal end of the small intestines, the abdominal pain would best be characterized as:
    A. "dull," with a gradual onset.
    B. "heavy," with a rapid onset.
    C. "burning," with a rapid onset.
    D. "crampy," with a slow onset.

38. Organs of the abdominal cavity are catagorized as:
    A. hollow, solid, and movable.
    B. vascular, solid, and hollow.
    C. fibrous, movable, and immovable.
    D. hollow, solid, and striated.

39. Rupture of which of the following abdominal structures would produce the fastest onset of hypoperfusion?
    A. descending aorta
    B. portal vein
    C. spleen
    D. liver

40. A person can live normally without which one of the following gastrointestinal organs?
    A. esophagus
    B. jejunum
    C. kidneys
    D. appendix

41. Which of the following is **not** a function of the skeletal system?

A. protection

B. support

C. mobility

D. reflexes

42. Another EMT-I tells you that a patient in a car accident has a possible fracture to the zygomatic arch. You would suspect that:

A. it involves the chin.

B. the patient may also have a black eye (periorbital ecchymosis).

C. the patient will need endotracheal intubation.

D. the patient has a lower extremity fracture.

43. Which of the following bones is **not** one found in the cranium?

A. parietal

B. temporal

C. acromion

D. frontal

44. The atlas and axis are part of:

A. the vertebral column.

B. the pelvis.

C. the thoracic rib cage.

D. the ankle joint.

45. Which of the following bones is **not** known as a long bone?

A. fibula

B. femur

C. humerus

D. sacrum

46. An injury to the metacarpals may affect the ability to:

A. walk.

B. write.

C. chew.

D. bend over.

47. Which of the following helps create smooth, pain-free movement?

A. articular cartilage

B. parietal fluid

C. greater omentum

D. arthroid discs

48. The vertebrae which must support the most weight are the:

A. cervical.

B. thoracic.

C. lumbar.

D. coccyx.

49. With a fracture of the humerus, what blood vessel may also be damaged?

A. radial artery

B. brachial artery

C. iliac artery

D. ulnar artery

50. The thoracic ribs offer protection to all the following organs, **except** the:

A. lungs.

B. diaphragm.

C. heart.

D. descending aorta.

51. Which of the following is primarily responsible for preventing the collapse of the alveoli?

A. visceral pleura

B. surfactant

C. parenchyma

D. pleural fluid

52. The posterior wall of the trachea is composed of:

A. cartilagenous rings.

B. branches of the terminal bronchioles.

C. lung parenchyma.

D. smooth muscle.

53. At which point do the bronchi enter the lungs?
    A. hilum
    B. pleura
    C. carina
    D. hyoid

54. Gas exchange can occur in all of the following areas, **except**:
    A. alveoli.
    B. alveolar ducts.
    C. pleura.
    D. terminal bronchioles.

55. The cricothyroid membrane is located:
    A. inferior to the thyroid cartilage and superior to the cricoid cartilage.
    B. superior to the thyroid cartilage and inferior to the hyoid bone.
    C. lateral to the cricoid and posterior to the trachea.
    D. inferior to the cricoid and superior to the thyroid cartilage.

56. The Hering-Breuer reflex is responsible for:
    A. monitoring blood flow through the pulmonary capillaries.
    B. preventing overexpansion of the lungs.
    C. decreasing respiratory rate due to increases in PaO_2.
    D. increasing myocardial contractility.

57. The majority of carbon dioxide is transported in the blood:
    A. attached to hemoglobin.
    B. dissolved in plasma.
    C. as bicarbonate.
    D. on the surface of the red blood cell.

58. Which of the following structures is primarily responsible for controlling expiration?

A. apneustic center
B. medullary chemoreceptors
C. cerebellar center
D. pneumotaxic center

59. The amount of dead space associated with ventilation in the adult male is approximately:
    A. 500 ml.
    B. 350 ml.
    C. 150 ml.
    D. 50 ml.

60. You have your patient on a nonrebreather mask at 15 lpm. You estimate the percentage of oxygen to be 95 percent. When calling in to the hospital, medical control asks what is the FiO_2. Which of the following would represent the FiO_2 in this patient?
    A. 95
    B. 1
    C. .5
    D. .95

61. A patient involved in a motor vehicle crash is unable to move his right lower extremity. He can feel both pain and light touch. The structure that was most likely injured is the:
    A. cerebellum.
    B. efferent nerve tract.
    C. parasympathetic nervous system.
    D. afferent nerve tract.

62. A patient faints while standing in line at the grocery store. The physician at the emergency department states that peripheral pooling caused her to faint. Which of the following is most likely responsible for the vasodilation leading to the fainting episode?
    A. efferent nerve tracts
    B. somatic nervous system

C. vagus nerve

D. cerebrum

63. What is acetylcholine?

A. The primary neurotransmitter of the parasympathetic nervous system.

B. A drug used to reduce edema in a spinal cord injured patient.

C. The substance found post-ganglionically in the sympathetic nervous system.

D. A substance that increases the heart rate and contraction.

64. A patient has apparently suffered a head injury. He has no fine motor coordination and is unable to maintain a posture. He most likely injured the:

A. cerebrum.

B. medulla oblongata.

C. mesencephalon.

D. cerebellum.

65. A patient has a fixed and dilated pupil. He most likely has an injury to which cranial nerve?

A. first

B. third

C. fifth

D. tenth

66. A hematoma that forms above the outer most layer of the meninges and below the skull is known as a(n):

A. subarachnoid hematoma.

B. epidural hematoma.

C. subdural hematoma.

D. intracerebral hematoma.

67. A person who was struck in the head has difficulty speaking. He has most likely suffered an injury to what portion of the brain?

A. occipital lobe

B. frontal lobe

C. parietal lobe

D. temporal lobe

68. The patient suffering from hypoglycemia typically presents with tachycardia; pale, cool, and clammy skin; and anxiousness. This is most likely caused by stimulation of the:

A. parasympathetic nervous system.

B. cerebellum.

C. sympathetic nervous system.

D. cerebrum.

69. Which part of the brain houses the hypothalmus?

A. cerebrum

B. diencephalon

C. mesencephalon

D. medulla

70. Which of the following responses would result from stimulation of an adrenergic fiber?

A. decreased heart rate

B. constricted pupil

C. increase in gastric motility

D. vasoconstriction

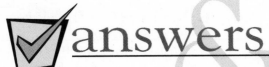
1.

B. Smooth muscle is contained within many internal organs. Through contraction, smooth muscle can bring about changes in size (pupils) or promote movement (digestion). Smooth muscle is found in the arterioles and functions to change the size of the lumen and thus regulates blood pressure. When the smooth muscle contracts, the lumen decreases in size and the blood pressure increases. Conversely, when the lumen increase in size the blood pressure is decreased. The structure of the heart is formed by cardiac muscle. Ligaments are responsible for connecting bone to bone. Skeletal muscle is responsible for promoting the movement of the skeleton, not smooth muscle.

2.

A. In light of the mechanism, location, and complaint of difficulty in moving the fingers, the EMT-Intermediate should consider a possible injury to the tendons that link the phalanges to the muscles in the forearm. Tendons connect muscle to bone. If the tendons on the back of the hand are severed, the link that provides for finger movement is greatly diminished or lost all together. Ligaments join bone to bone at joints.

3.

D. For skeletal muscle to facilitate movement, the individual muscle fibers must contract. When muscle fibers contract, they shorten and exert a pulling motion—thereby initiating movement. Skeletal muscles cannot promote movement by a pushing motion, for when they push, relaxation occurs.

4.

C. A prime function of the human muscular system is to provide movement via the manipulation of the skeletal bones. The bones do not move themselves, but rely on the skeletal muscles. Therefore, the skeletal system provides the body with structure and the muscular system provides the movement. Internal fluid loss is more a function of the skin rather than the skeletal muscle, and fat is stored by adipose tissue and not the actual muscle cells.

5.

B. Because field distinguishment of strains, sprains, dislocation, and fractures is difficult, appropriate EMT-Intermediate treatment would include the "worst case scenario," assumption of a fracture and subsequent immobilization. Immobilizing a knee in the position found can effectively be accomplished with a vacuum splint or a soft splint such as a pillow and tape. In this situation, compression bandages are ill advised in that they do not allow for outward expansion of edema. Restricting this naturally occurring injury response could cause inward compression of blood vessels and nerve fibers and a general worsening of the situation. Application of ice is appropriate in the management of the edema, but does not represent overall best choice since the injury demands immobilization also. The same holds true for transporting in a position of comfort.

6.

B. Within the human body, the kidneys serve to cleanse waste products from the blood. The hypothalamus regulates body temperature, while glucose absorption and feces production generally occur in the gastrointestinal system.

7.

D. Based upon anatomical location, the EMT-Intermediate must suspect possible damage to the left kidney. The kidneys are located in the retroperitoneal cavity between the 12th thoracic and 3rd lumbar vertebrae. Any blunt trauma to the back with an associated rib fracture must raise the index of suspicion as to kidney involvement. The bladder is located in the pelvic cavity and would not be affected by a blow to the back. Also, the liver is located on the right side of the peritoneal cavity, not the left. The stomach is also located in the peritoneal cavity but in front of the kidneys.

8.

C. From the internal to external environment, urine must pass through the kidney, ureter, bladder, and urethra.

9.

A. The urinary bladder is located low in the pelvic cavity, directly behind the pubic bone. The vertebral column lies posterior to the bladder. The urinary bladder is not located in the abdominal cavity.

10.

B. Kidneys facilitate the formation of urine. Acute renal failure would cause a decrease in the formation and output of urine. An increase in urinary output would not be noted. Vomiting of blood and blood in the stool arise from the intestinal tract and are not directly related to acute renal failure.

11.

C. In the male reproductive system, the testes are responsible for the production of sperm and the secretion of hormones.

12.

B. Testosterone is synthesized from cholesterol in the testes and is the primary hormone of the male reproductive system.

13.

A. The female reproductive system is comprised of the ovaries, uterus, and the vagina.

14.

A. The primary female sex hormone is estrogen.

15.

D. The placenta is the organ responsible for the exchange of oxygen and nutrients between maternal and fetal circulation.

16.

B. The pituitary gland is the endocrine organ known as the "master gland" because it secretes several hormones that control other endocrine glands.

17.

D. Oxytocin is the hormone which enhances uterine contraction and stimulates milk production in the mammary glands. It is secreted by the posterior pituitary gland.

18.

A. Epinephrine and norepinephrine are sympathomimetic hormones produced by the medulla of the adrenal glands. Their effects include increasing blood pressure by increasing heart rate, strength of contraction, and constricting peripheral blood vessels.

19.

C. Although the interactions of the pancreatic hormones are not completely understood, glucagon and insulin work in opposition to each other. Glucagon increases the blood glucose level by releasing glucose stores in the liver, while insulin decreases it by aiding its entry into the cells.

20.

C. Inadequate production of insulin causes diabetes mellitus. It is a common metabolic disorder leading to a chronic elevation in blood glucose levels.

21.

D. The right atrium receives deoxygenated blood from the body by way of the superior and inferior vena cava. The blood is then moved to the right ventricle by atrial contraction and gravity. The right ventricle perfuses the blood through the lungs for oxygenation. After being received by the left atrium and delivered to the left ventricle, it is pumped to the body.

22.

A. Chordae tendonae are fibrous structures that are attached to papillary muscles in the ventricles. Their purpose is to prevent regurgitation of blood into the atria that would occur if the AV valves were allowed to invert during ventricular contraction. There are no such structures in the atria nor on the semilunar valves.

23.

B. The cardiac cells have four special properties which are unique only to the cells of the heart. These properties include conductivity, the ability to propagate an electrical impulse from cell to cell; automaticity, the ability to initiate its own impulse; contractility, the ability to contract when stimulated; and excitability, the ability to respond to an impulse.

24.

B. Blood flow through the heart starts at the right atrium, and then proceeds through the right ventricle and pulmonary arteries, to the lungs. Blood returns from the lungs via the pulmonary veins and enters the left atrium which delivers it to the left ventricle and then to the aorta.

25.

A. The heart uses the diastole phase for filling, which in turn provides the preload for the ventricles. In situations of extreme tachycardia, the diastolic period is so short that there is ineffective filling, which subsequently drops ventricular stroke volume. The increased heart rate will increase O_2 requirements of the heart, and diminish coronary artery perfusion since they are perfused during the diastolic phase.

26.

B. A drug which makes the heart contract more forcefully, also known as a positive inotropic agent, will increase the stroke volume of the heart. This increase in stroke volume also increases cardiac output. To increase the rate, one would have to administer a sympathomimetic or parasympatholytic. An increase in systemic vascular resistance is achieved by giving an alpha stimulating drug.

27.

A. The primary pacemaker of the heart is the sinoatrial or SA node. It has an intrinsic discharge rate of 60 to 100 beats per minute. The intra-atrial pathways only distribute the discharge wave for uniform atrial contraction. The AV node is the secondary pacemaker with a discharge rate of 40 to 60 beats per minute. The bundle of His transmits the impulse from the AV node to the bundle branches.

28.

C. Dopaminergic receptors are in the renal vessels and mesenteric vasculature. Stimulation or blockage of these sites will influence the degree of constriction or dilation they experience. Influencing either the sympathetic or parasympathetic (vagal) nervous system will alter the heart rate.

29.

C. Inotropic agents increase the force of contraction in the ventricles. A positive dromotropic agent increases conduction velocity and a chronotropic agent increases heart rate. Isotropic is a fabricated term.

30.

C. The bicuspid valve, also known as the mitral valve, is located between the left ventricle and left atrium. It is under the greatest amount of strain caused by pressures generated during left ventricular contraction. In some patients, this valve progressively fails allowing regurgitation of blood into the left atrium, increasing hydrostatic pressure in the pulmonary veins and eventually leading to pulmonary edema.

31.

D. The adrenal glands sit atop each kidney and release hormones into the blood stream from autonomic stimulation. The pancreas secretes certain digestive enzymes. The stomach helps with the digestion of food. The rectum is part of the distal GI tract leading to elimination of fecal material from the body.

32.

A. The pancreas is a gland with two major purposes. It creates hormones for the body to help regulate glucose levels (endocrine role), and it also produces digestive enzymes for the body (exocrine role). The liver stores glycogen, not the pancreas, and bile is produced by the liver. Estrogen is a female hormone secreted by the ovaries.

33.

B. From the stomach, food passes into the small intestine for continued digestion and absorption of necessary contents. The small intestine is comprised of three parts (in order): duodenum, jejunum, and ileum. The ascending colon is a portion of the large intestine.

34.

A. The wave-like contractions that result in the propulsion of food through the alimentary tract are known as peristalsis. Paresis is weakness of voluntary muscle and portal waves does not mean anything. Muscular intropy would refer to stimulation or contraction of a muscle.

35.

C. The gall bladder is located inferior to the liver, and stores bile created by the liver. The urinary bladder stores urine until it is eliminated from the body.

36.

B. Gastric ulceration occurs when the hydrochloric acid of the stomach erodes the mucosal lining of the stomach wall. This can be severe enough to cause gastric hemorrhaging. Gastritis may present with similar discomfort as gastric ulceration, but it refers specifically to inflammation of the mucosal lining. Diverticulitis is an inward pouching of intestinal tissue, usually located in the large intestine and is a common cause of hematochezia.

37.

C. The small intestine is usually acidic because of the hydrochloric acid which comes from the stomach during the digestion process. If perforation should occur, the low pH of the contents usually causes immediate pain of a burning characteristic as the acid acts on the other abdominal structures.

38.

B. Organs of the abdominal cavity can be categorized into hollow organs (stomach, intestines, gall bladder, etc.), solid organs (spleen, liver, pancreas), or vascular organs (vena cava, aorta). This categorization is useful because organs in the same category typically have similar presentations should an injury occur.

39.

A. The descending aorta is a vascular structure that provides arterial blood to the abdominal organs and lower extremities. Should a rupture occur, it can cause massive hemorrhaging, as the blood will exit the aorta under systolic pressure. This will produce the fastest onset of hypoperfusion of the structures listed.

40.

D. The appendix is a structure located at the junction of the small and large intestine in the right lower quadrant. It is not uncommon for it to be removed when it ruptures or becomes inflamed, and it has no effect of quality of life.

41.

D. The skeletal system provides three very important functions: support, protection to organs within certain cavities (for example, the cranium or thoracic cavity), and motion in conjunction with muscles. It does not play a role in reflex arcs. These are a function of the nervous system.

42.

B. The zygomatic arch is commonly known as the cheekbone. Given its location, a fracture of the zygomatic arch may also result in small hemorrhages into the soft tissue around the eye and result in a black eye. The bone in the chin is known as the mandible. Intubation needs and lower extremity findings may be present if it is significant trauma, but is not dependent on zygomatic fractures.

43.

C. The cranium is created by the fusion of numerous bones. The major bones are the frontal bone, the temporal bones, the occipital bone, and the parietal bones. The acromion is the process located at the junction of the scapula and clavicle.

44.

A. The atlas is the first cervical vertebrae and it supports the skull. It allows the rotation movement characteristic to the head. The second cervical vertebrae is known as the axis, and has a protrusion, the ondontoid process, which projects into the atlas and allows the vertebrae to remain aligned. They both are part of the vertebral column.

45.

D. The sacrum is a bone that is part of the pelvic structure, and is considered to be an irregular bone. The other three bones are considered long bones.

46.

B. Metacarpals are the smaller bones of the hands. An injury here would most likely result in an inability to use the fingers or to write. The metatarsals are small foot bones which could cause inability to walk. Damage to the mandible can cause an inability to chew. Vertebral damage could result in an inability to bend over.

47.

A. The articular surface is a smooth cartilage which overlays the point where two bones move over each other. This greatly reduces friction and pain associated with bones rubbing. Synovial fluid is a lubricating fluid present in the joint capsules. The greater omentum is a lining in the abdominal cavity that helps protect the abdominal contents.

48.

C. The lumbar vertebrae have the largest body section, which is the portion that supports weight.

49.

B. The brachial artery travels along the humerus. Alongside every bone is a nerve, artery, and vein. In most locations in the body the name of the bone is also the name of the artery, i.e., the radial artery runs along side the radius.

50.

D. The sternum, ribs, and thoracic vertebrae provide protection to the lungs, heart, and diaphragm along with other thoracic structures. They do not, however, protect the descending aorta since it travels through the abdominal cavity—beyond the level of the ribs.

51.

B. Surfactant is a lipoprotein that decreases the surface tension of the alveoli and prevents collapse.

52.

D. The posterior wall of the trachea is only comprised of smooth muscle. The anterior and lateral aspects are supported by cartilagenous structures.

53.

A. The hilum is the point where the bronchi enter the lungs.

54.

C. Gas exchange will occur primarily in the alveoli, however, minimal exchange may occur in the alveolar ducts and terminal bronchioles. No gas exchange occurs in the pleura.

55.

A. The cricothyroid membrane is located inferior to the thyroid cartilage and superior to the cricoid cartilage.

56.

B. The Hering-Breuer reflex is responsible for preventing overexpansion of the lungs. Stretch fibers located in the lung send impulses to the medulla to regulate the volume of air taken into the lungs.

57.

C. About 66 percent of the circulating carbon dioxide is transported in the form of bicarbonate (HCO_3). To a much lesser extent, CO_2 is transported dissolved in plasma and attached to hemoglobin.

58.

D. The pneumotaxic center, located in the pons, is responsible for controlling expiration. The apneustic center, also located in the pons, is the backup to stimulate breathing if the respiratory center in the medulla would fail.

59.

C. The amount of dead space associated with ventilation is about 150 ml in the adult male patient. Thus, 350 ml of the typical tidal volume of 500 ml is used in gas exchange.

60.

D. FiO_2 is the fraction of inspired oxygen. The FiO_2 is 0.95 if the patient is breathing in 95 percent oxygen. An FiO_2 of 1.0 represents a patient breathing 100 percent oxygen.

61.

B. Efferent nerve tracts transmit impulses from the brain to muscle and control motor function.

62.

C. The parasympathetic nervous system affects vasodilation. About 75 percent of the parasympathetic nervous impulses are carried by the vagus nerve.

63.

A. Acetylcholine is the neurotransmitter of the parasympathetic nervous system. The neurotransmitter of the sympathetic nervous system is norepinehprine.

64.

D. The cerebellum is responsible for controlling fine motor movement, coordination, posture, and equilibrium.

65.

B. The third cranial nerve (occulomotor nerve) controls the pupillary response.

66.

B. The space between the dura mater, the outermost layer of the meninges, and the skull is called the epidural space. A collection of blood in this space is called an epidural hematoma.

67.

D. The temporal lobe area would control speech. The parietal area controls sensory, occipital controls vision, and the frontal lobe controls personality and motor function.

68.

C. The sympathetic nervous system, known as the "fight or flight" response, will increase heart rate, and cause the skin to become pale, cool, and clammy in the hypoglycemic patient. This is a response from the secretion and circulation of epinephrine.

69.

B. The hypothalmus, thalmus, and limbic system are all housed in the diencephalon.

70.

D. An adrenergic fiber is usually associated with the sympathetic nervous system. Vasoconstriction is a sympathetic nervous system response.

Appendix: D.O.T. Objectives

CHAPTER 1: ROLES AND RESPONSIBILITIES

Upon completion of this chapter, the student will be able to:

1.1.1 Identify and describe those activities performed by an EMT-Intermediate in the field.

1.1.2 Define the role of the EMT-Intermediate.

1.1.3 Describe and contrast the difference between an EMT-Ambulance and EMT-Intermediate training program.

1.1.4 Define the terms "ethics" and "professionalism."

1.1.5 Describe the differences between ethical behavior and legal requirements.

1.1.6 State specific activities that are most appropriate to ethical behavior.

1.1.7 Identify whether a particular activity is unethical and/or illegal, given certain patient care situations.

1.1.8 Identify whether a particular activity is ethical or unethical given certain patient care situations.

1.1.9 Define the term "professional."

1.1.10 Define the term "health care professional."

1.1.11 Identify whether a particular activity is professional or unprofessional given certain patient care situations.

1.1.12 State certain activities that are most appropriate to professional behavior.

1.1.13 List current state requirements for EMT-Intermediate continuing education.

1.1.14 Define and discuss at least three reasons why continuing education is important for the EMT-Intermediate.

1.1.15 Define the terms "certification," "licensure," and "registration."

1.1.16 Name and describe current state legislation outlining the scope of prehospital advanced life support.

1.1.17 State the reason it is important to keep one's EMT-Intermediate certification current.

1.1.18 State the major purposes of a national association.

1.1.19 State the major purposes of a national registration agency.

1.1.20 State the major benefits of subscribing to professional journals.

1.1.21 State the benefits of EMT-Intermediates teaching in the community.

CHAPTER 2: EMS SYSTEMS

Upon completion of this chapter, the student will be able to:

1.2.1 Discuss citizen access and the various mechanisms of obtaining it.

1.2.2 Discuss prehospital care as an extension of hospital care.

1.2.3 Define stabilization of patients.

1.2.4 Define and describe medical control.

1.2.5 Describe physician responsibility for medical control.

1.2.6 Describe the relationship between the physician on the scene, the EMT-I, and the physician on the radio.
   a. Physician who is with the patient when the EMT-I arrives
   b. Physician who arrives on the scene after the EMT-Is have started evaluating and treating the patient

1.2.7 Describe the benefits of EMT-I follow-up on patient condition, diagnosis, and retrospective review of prehospital care.

1.2.8 Describe GSA/KKK ambulance standards.

1.2.9 Define the American College of Surgeons' Essential Equipment List and how it relates to local and state laws.

1.2.10 Define the national standard levels of prehospital provider as defined by the curriculum, respectively.
   a. Discuss ambulance placement and the parameters that should be utilized in its development, including the differences in urban, suburban, and rural settings.

1.2.11 Discuss the medical community role in overseeing prehospital care.

1.2.12 Define protocols and standing orders.

1.2.13 Describe the development of protocols.

1.2.14 Define local training standards.

1.2.15 Describe the legislation in the EMT-I's state in regard to prehospital care.

1.2.16 Describe integration of prehospital care into the continuum of total patient care with the emergency department phase of hospital care.

1.2.17 Discuss replacement of equipment and supplies.

1.2.18 Discuss the EMT-I's initial responsibilities when arriving on the scene.

1.2.19 Describe the relationship between the physician on the radio and the EMT-I at the scene.

1.2.20 Discuss the varying philosophies between the management of medical patients and trauma patients, prehospital.

1.2.21 Describe the transition of patient care from the EMT-I, including:
 a. Transfer of responsibility (legal and medical)
 b. Reporting of patient status to physician or nurse

1.2.22 Describe the ability of physician-run critique based on documentation.

1.2.23 Describe retrospective evaluation of patient care, including run report review, continuing education, skill practice, and skill deterioration.

CHAPTER 3: MEDICAL/LEGAL CONSIDERATIONS

Upon completion of this chapter, the student will be able to:

1.3.1 Discuss the significance and scope of the following in relation to EMT practice.
 a. State Medical Practice Act
 b. Good Samaritan Act/Civil Immunity
 c. State EMS statutes
 d. State motor vehicle codes
 e. State and local guidelines for "Do Not Resuscitate."

1.3.2 Define the following:
 a. Negligence
 b. Medical liability
 c. Tort
 d. Duty to act
 e. Battery
 f. Slander
 g. Informed consent
 h. Expressed consent
 i. Implied consent
 j. Abandonment
 k. Liable
 l. Assault
 m. False imprisonment

1.3.3 Describe the significance of accurate documentation and record keeping in substantiating incidents.

1.3.4 Identify situations that require the EMT-I to report those incidents to appropriate authorities.

1.3.5 Describe the four elements to prove medical liability.

1.3.6 Describe the significance of obtaining expressed consent.

1.3.7 Describe the extent to which force and restraint may be used to protect the EMT, the patient, and the third party.

CHAPTER 4: MEDICAL TERMINOLOGY

Upon completion of this chapter, the student will be able to:

1.4.1 Define and contrast medical terms.

1.4.2 Identify various medical terms given one or more anatomical parts of the body.

1.4.3 Identify common medical abbreviations.

1.4.4 Identify common root words and determine their meanings.

1.4.5 Identify and define common prefixes and suffixes.

1.4.6 Locate one or more medical terms in a medical dictionary.

CHAPTER 5: EMS COMMUNICATIONS

Upon completion of this chapter, the student will be able to:

1.5.1 Describe the phases of communications necessary to complete a typical EMS event.

1.5.2 Name the possible components of an EMS communications system and explain the function of each.

1.5.3 Describe maintenance procedures for the field radio equipment.

1.5.4 Describe the position of the antenna on a portable transmitter/receiver that will deliver maximum coverage.

1.5.5 Describe an advantage of a repeater system over a non-repeater system.

1.5.6 Describe basic functions and responsibilities of the Federal Communications Commission (FCC).

1.5.7 Describe the responsibilities of an EMS dispatcher.

1.5.8 Name information items that must be gathered from a caller by the dispatcher.

1.5.9 Describe the ten-code used in the local community (optional).

1.5.10 Describe three communications techniques that influence the clarity of radio transmissions.

1.5.11 Describe three communications techniques that influence the content of radio transmissions.

1.5.12 Describe the importance of written medical protocols.

1.5.13 Describe two purposes of verbal communication of patient information to the hospital.

1.5.14 Describe information that should be included in patient assessment information verbally reported to the physician.

1.5.15 Organize a list of patient assessment information in the correct order for radio transmission to the physician according to the format used locally.

1.5.16 Name five uses of the EMS run form.

S1.5.17 Demonstrate the proper use of a mobile transmitter/receiver to receive and transmit information.

S1.5.18 Demonstrate the proper use of a portable transmitter/receiver to receive and transmit information.

S1.5.19 Demonstrate the proper use of a digital encoder.

S1.5.20 Demonstrate the proper use of a mobile or portable transmitter in a real or simulated patient situation to organize and transmit patient assessment information, using a standardized format.

S1.5.21 Properly complete a written EMS for based on a real or simulated patient situation.

CHAPTER 6: GENERAL PATIENT ASSESSMENT AND INITIAL MANAGEMENT

Upon completion of this chapter, the student will be able to:

1.6.1 Establish priorities of care based on threat-to-life conditions.

1.6.2 Describe the four phases of patient assessment.

1.6.3 Discuss the possible environmental hazards that the EMT-I may encounter and the means of protecting him/her in this environment.

1.6.4 Describe the environmental hazards which a patient might encounter.

1.6.5 Describe the problems and EMT-I might encounter in a hostile situation and describe mechanisms of management.

1.6.6 Describe the various types of protective equipment available to the EMT-I for self-protection and patient protection.

1.6.7 Discuss the appropriate methods of patient protection in each situation.

1.6.8 Discuss backup personnel, transportation, and equipment.

1.6.9 Define and describe the various classifications of emergencies which an EMT-I will encounter. Base this on medical needs.

1.6.10 Describe the primary survey and what areas are critical to evaluate.

1.6.11 Describe the anatomy of the following: upper airway, tongue, hypopharynx, nasopharynx, oropharynx, larynx, vocal cords.

1.6.12 Describe the function of the vocal cords.

1.6.13 Describe the flow of air from outside the body into the trachea.

1.6.14 Describe the reasons for and mechanism of humidification and warming of the air as it passes through the naso- and oropharynx.

1.6.15 Describe the pathological conditions that can occur in the nose, pharynx, and larynx to obstruct or retard air flow and identify the complications of laryngeal fracture.

1.6.16 Describe the methods of airway management.

1.6.17 Describe the methods and management of an obstructed airway.

1.6.18 Describe the mechanical methods of airway management (oral, nasal, and EOA) including the benefits and limitations.

1.6.19 Describe how the cervical spine is protected throughout these maneuvers.

1.6.20 Describe the anatomy of the following:
   a. Lungs
   b. Trachea
   c. Alveolus
   d. Diaphragm
   e. Thoracic wall
   f. Pleural space

1.6.21 Describe how pulmonary ventilation (inhalation and exhalation) is accomplished.

1.6.22 Describe the gaseous exchange across the alveoli-capillary membrane (O_2 and CO_2)

1.6.23 Describe the pulmonary problems that can complicate exhalation and inhalation, the mechanisms by which they reduce ventilation, and management of each problem, including
   a. Open pneumothorax
   b. Diaphragmatic injury
   c. Closed pneumothorax
   d. Flail chest

1.6.24 Describe the problems of ventilation.

1.6.25 Define mouth-to-mask ventilation, its benefits and limitations.

1.6.26 Discuss the bag-valve-mask (BVM), its benefits and limitations.

1.6.27 Discuss the techniques for evaluating the effectiveness of ventilation.

1.6.28 Describe the anatomy of the heart and cardiovascular system.

1.6.29 Describe the problems that occur with decreased perfusion.

1.6.30 Describe the pathophysiology of cardiac arrest.

1.6.31 Describe the mechanisms of evaluating the effectiveness of perfusion, including pulse, skin color, capillary refill.

1.6.32 Descuss ventilation with an EOA.

1.6.33 Discuss ventilation with an endotracheal tube (optional).

1.6.34 Describe the equipment and method of suctioning the airway, pharynx, and endotrachael tube (optional).

1.6.35 Describe the anatomy of the skin, bones, vessels, and subcutaneous tissue as it relates to hemorrhage control.

1.6.36 Discuss the benefits and complications of hemorrhage control by the following means:
   a. Direct pressure
   b. Tourniquets
   c. Hemostats

1.6.37 Define a mini-neurological examination (level of consciousness).

1.6.38 Describe exposing the patient's body for total evaluation.

1.6.39 Discuss when this should and should not be carried out.

1.6.40 Define shock.

1.6.41 Describe the reasons for and mechanisms of patient reassessment in the resuscitation phase.

1.6.42 Define the components of secondary survey and its benefits for patient evaluation.

1.6.43 Describe the assessment of the head, neck, thorax, abdomen, extremities, and nervous system.

1.6.44 Describe the trauma score and define its usefulness and how it is accomplished.

1.6.45 Discuss the important components that must be identified in taking an appropriate history from a patient.

1.6.46 Describe the laboratory samples that are drawn in the field when the IV is started and their usefulness.

1.6.47 Define the definitive care phase.

1.6.48 Describe how a patient is packaged and stabilized for transportation to the hospital, including airway ventilation, IV fluids, pneumatic antishock garment, fracture stabilization, and bandaging.

1.6.49 Describe how the patient is immobilized to the backboard.

1.6.50 Describe how the patient is immobilized to the stretcher and to the ambulance.

1.6.51 Describe patient extrication.

1.6.52 Describe how the patient is monitored en route to the hospital.

1.6.53 Describe how the hospitals are selected for receipt of patients based on patient need and hospital capability.

1.6.54 Describe the benefits and complications of lights and sirens and when they should be used.

1.6.55 Describe the interaction of the EMT-I and medical command authority in regard to receiving hospital, family physician on the scene, bystander physician on the scene, orders for patient care, needs of the family, and needs of the patient.

1.6.56 Describe the usefulness of a run report.

1.6.57 Describe the mechanisms of continued evaluation of the patient en route to the hospital.

S1.6.58 Perform a rapid assessment of the patient to identify priorities for care.

S1.6.59 Demonstrate the assessment of the head, neck, thorax, abdomen, extremities, and neurological system.

S1.6.60 Demonstrate effective mouth-to-mask ventilation.

S1.6.61 Demonstrate effective bag-valve-
   a. mask
   b. EOA
   c. ET (optional)

S1.6.62 Demonstrate effective cardiopulmonary resuscitation.

S1.6.63 Demonstrate the manual methods of airway management.

S1.6.64 Demonstrate the methods of management of an obstructed airway.

S1.6.65 Demonstrate the mechanical methods of airway management
   a. Nasal
   b. Oral
   c. EOA
   d. ET (optional)

S1.6.66 Demonstrate the use of self-protection equipment such as an air pack (breathing apparatus).

S1.6.67 Demonstrate the use of various types of portable and fixed suction devices.

CHAPTER 7: AIRWAY MANAGEMENT AND VENTILATION

Upon completion of this chapter, the student will be able to:

1.7.1 Describe the anatomy of the mouth, hypopharynx, trachea, larynx.

1.7.2 Describe the relationship between:
   a. Cords and larynx
   b. Esophagus and larynx
   c. Epiglottis and larynx
   d. Tongue and larynx
   e. True cords and false cords
   f. Pharynx and larynx

1.7.3 Given a list of arterial oxygen concentrations, the student should be able to select the normal PO_2 for a young adult breathing air.

1.7.4 Given a list of arterial carbon dioxide concentrations, the student should be able to select the normal PCO_2.

1.7.5 Given an increase in arterial PCO_2, the student should be able to name this condition and describe its effect on respiratory activity and on blood pH in the normal individual.

1.7.6 Given a decrease in arterial PCO_2, the student should be able to name this condition and describe its effect on respiratory activity and on blood pH in the normal individual.

1.7.7 Given an increase in CO_2 production, the student should be able to list at least two ways in which this increase may occur.

1.7.8 Given an increase in CO_2 elimination, the student should be able to describe how this elimination can occur.

1.7.9 Given a list of statements, the student should be able to identify the statement that best describes the purpose of suctioning a patient.

1.7.10 Given a diagram of a piston-powered suction unit, the student should be able to label and describe the operation and cleaning of each component and attached part.

1.7.11 Given that there are various types of suction units, the student should be able to list at least four different types of units determined by the method in which the suction effect is obtained.

1.7.12 Given that there are various types of suction catheters, the student should be able to list at least three different types, determined by difference in use and material composition.

1.7.13 Given a list of situations describing patients who require suctioning, the student should indicate which type of catheter should be used.

1.7.14 Given a list of statements, the student should be able to identify the statement that best describes the purpose of using the esophageal obturator airway.

1.7.15 Given a list of situations describing patients with airway maintenance problems or potential airway maintenance problems, the student should be able to identify situations in which the use of the esophageal obturator airway is indicated and contraindicatied.

1.7.16 Given a list of situations, the student should be able to identify those situations in which the esophageal airway may be removed.

1.7.17 Given a list of advantages, the student should be able to identify the advantages of using the esophageal obturator airway over other methods of airway control.

1.7.18 Given a list of airway adjuncts, advantages and disadvantages, the student should be able to match the airway adjuncts with the advantages and disadvantages.

1.7.19 Given an adult mannequin, oropharyngeal and nasopharyngeal airways, pocket mask, oxygen cylinder, and bag-valve-mask, the student should be able to demonstrate the procedure for administering intermittent positive pressure ventilation using:
   a. Pocket mask
   b. Bag-valve-mask and oropharyngeal airway
   c. Bag-valve-mask with oxygen
   d. Nasopharyngeal aiway with bag-valve-mask

S1.7.20 Given a bag-valve-mask, the student should be able to demonstrate the assembly, disassembly, and cleaning of the bag-valve-mask unit.

S1.7.21 Given an adult mannequin, an oropharyngeal airway, and a demand-valve unit, the student should be able to demonstrate the procedure for performing intermittent positive-pressure ventilation.

S1.7.22 Given a demand-valve unit, the student should be able to demonstrate the assembly, disassembly, and cleaning of the unit.

1.7.23 Given a list of disadvantages, the student should be able to identify the disadvantages of using the esophageal obturator airway over other methods of airway control.

1.7.24 Given a diagram of the esophageal obturator airway, the student should be able to label and describe the function of all component parts.

1.7.25 Given a list of equipment and materials, the student should be able to identify those items that must be available before esophageal obturation is begun.

1.7.26 Given that a patient requires an esophageal obturator airway, the student should be able to list the procedures for insertion of the esophageal airway, including all steps in the proper sequence.

1.7.27 Given a list of errors, the student should be able to identify common errors in the use of the esophageal airway.

1.7.28 Describe laryngoscope, suction, endotracheal tube and bag-valve-mask (optional).

1.7.29 Discuss indications and contraindications of endotracheal intubation (optional).

1.7.30 Discuss alternatives to endotracheal intubation (optional).

1.7.31 Discuss skill deterioration and methods of prevention (optional).

1.7.32 Discuss need for rapid placement of ET tube (optional).

1.7.33 Discuss methods of assuring and maintaining correct placement of ET tube (optional).

1.7.34 Given that a patient needs suctioning and already has an endotracheal tube in place, the student should be able to describe the difference between endotracheal suctioning and oropharyngeal suctioning, including: (optional)
   a. Dangers
   b. Precautions

S1.7.35 Given an adult intubation mannequin, an esophageal obturator airway, 30-cc syringe, and a bag-valve unit, the student should be able to demonstrate the technique for the insertion of an esophageal obturator airway. He/She should further be able to demonstrate endotracheal intubation with the esophageal obturator in place and subsequent correct removal of the obturator (optional).

S1.7.36 Demonstrate placement of an ET within 45 seconds (optional).

S1.7.37 Demonstrate ventilation with bag valve and endotracheal tube (optional).

S1.7.38 Demonstrate method by assuring and maintaining correct placement of ET tube (optional).

S1.7.39 Demonstrate reventilation for missed intubation (optional).

S1.7.40 Demonstrate skills described above both on mannequin and a live patient (optional).

CHAPTER 8: ASSESSMENT AND MANAGEMENT OF SHOCK

Upon completion of this chapter, the student will be able to:

1.8.1 Define shock based on aerobic and anaerobic metabolism.

1.8.2 Discuss the prevention of anaerobic metabolism.

1.8.3 Discuss red blood cell oxygenation in the lungs based on alveolar O_2 levels and transportation across the alveolar capillary wall.

1.8.4 Discuss tissue oxygenation based on tissue perfusion and release of oxygen.

1.8.5 Discuss the role played by respiration and inadequate ventilation in the management of shock.

1.8.6 Describe perfusion and the mechanisms to improve cardiac output based on the strength and rate of contractions.

1.8.7 Discuss the fluid component of the cardiovascular system and the relationship between the volume of the fluid and the size of the container.

1.8.8 Discuss systemic vascular resistance, the relationship of diastolic pressure to the SVR, and the effect of diastolic pressure on coronary circulation.

1.8.9 Discuss the container size in relation to the fluid volume and the effect on blood returning to the heart.

1.8.10 Discuss body fluids based on total body water, intracellular fluid, and extracellular fluid.

1.8.11 Identify the significant anions and cations in the body.

1.8.12 Describe the role of protein.

1.8.13 Discuss osmosis. Define semi-permeable membranes and discuss their function.

1.8.14 Define isotonic fluids, hypotonic fluids, and hypertonic fluids.

1.8.15 Define and discuss diffusion.

1.8.16 Define active transport.

1.8.17 Describe the mechanisms of concentration of electrolytes.

1.8.18 Define acid-base balance.

1.8.19 Discuss acid-base balance based on hydrogenion concentration, pH, and buffer systems.

1.8.20 Define and discuss the following:
   a. Respiratory acidosis
   b. Respiratory alkalosis
   c. Metabolic acidosis
   d. Metabolic alkalosis

1.8.21 Describe the mechanism of the body response to perfusion change.

1.8.22 Identify the role of the baroreceptor.

1.8.23 Describe how the actions of the baroreceptor affect blood pressure and perfusion.

1.8.24 Describe compensated shock.

1.8.25 Describe uncompensated shock, both cardiac and peripheral effects.

1.8.26 Discuss the assessment of the patient's perfusion status, based on physical observations within the primary survey, including pulse, skin temperature, and capillary refill.

1.8.27 Discuss the relationship of the neurological exam to assessment of hypoperfusion and oxygenation.

1.8.28 Describe the information provided by the following in physical examination: pulse, blood pressure, diastolic pressure, systolic pressure, skin color, appearance, temperature and respiration.

1.8.29 Discuss management of a shocky patient. Include red cell oxygenation, tissue ischemic sensitivity, IV fluids, and the pneumatic antishock garment.

1.8.30 Describe the beneficial and detrimental effects of the pneumatic antishock garment.

1.8.31 Describe the indication and contraindications for the pneumatic anitshock garment.

1.8.32 Discuss fluid replacement, the types of fluid that are available, and the benefits and detrimental effects of each.

1.8.33 Discuss how fluid replacement is monitored and controlled.

1.8.34 Discuss the routes of fluid replacement and the advantages and disadvantages of each.

S1.8.35 Demonstrate in order of priority the steps of shock resuscitation.

S1.8.36 Demonstrate the use of the pneumatic antishock garment.

S1.8.37 Demonstrate the proper technique to insert an intravenous catheter.

CHAPTER 9: DEFIBRILLATION

Upon completion of this chapter, the student will be able to:

1.9.1 Describe the size, shape and location/orientation (in regard to other body structures) of the heart muscle.

1.9.2 Identify the location of the following structures on a diagram of the normal heart:

a. Pericardium
b. Myocardium
c. Epicardium
d. Right and left atria
e. Interatrial septum
f. Right and left ventricles
g. Intraventricular septum
h. Superior and inferior vena cava
i. Aorta
j. Pulmonary vessels
k. Coronary arteries
l. Tricispid valve
m. Mitral valve
n. Aortic valve
o. Pulmonary valve
p. Papillary muscles
q. Chordae tendonae

1.9.3 Describe the function of each structure listed in Objective 1.9.2.

1.9.4 Describe the distribution of the coronary arteries and the parts of the heart supplied by each artery.

1.9.5 Differentiate the structural and functional aspects of arterial and venous blood vessels.

1.9.6 Define the following terms that refer to cardiac physiology:
a. Stroke volume
b. Starling's Law
c. Preload
d. Afterload
e. Cardiac output
f. Blood pressure

1.9.7 Describe the electrical properties of the heart.

1.9.8 Describe the normal sequence of electrical conduction through the heart and state the purpose of this conduction system.

1.9.9 Describe the location and function of the following structures of the electrical conduction system:
a. SA node
b. Internodal and interatrial tracts
c. AV node
d. Bundle of His
e. Bundle branches
f. Purkinje fibers

1.9.10 Define cardiac depolarization and describe the major electrolyte changes that occur in each process.

1.9.11 Describe an ECG.

1.9.12 Define the following terms as they relate to the electrical activity of the heart:
a. Isoelectric line

b. QRS complex
c. P wave

1.9.13 Name the common chief complaints of cardiac patients.

1.9.14 Describe why the following occur in patients with cardiac problems:
a. Chest pain or discomfort
b. Shoulder, arm, neck, or jaw pain/discomfort
c. Dyspnea
d. Syncope
e. Palpitations/abnormal heartbeat

1.9.15 Describe those questions to be asked during history taking for each of the common cardiac chief complaints.

1.9.16 Describe the four most pertinent aspects of the past medical history in a patient with a suspected cardiac problem.

1.9.17 Describe those aspects of the physical examination that should be given special attention in the patient with suspected cardiac problems.

1.9.18 Describe the significance of the following physical exam findings in a cardiac patient:
a. Altered level of consciousness
b. Peripheal edema
c. Cyanosis
d. Poor capillary refill
e. Cool, clammy skin

1.9.19 State the numerical values assigned to each small and each large box on the ECG graph paper for each axis.

1.9.20 Define ECG artifact and name the causes.

1.9.21 State the steps in the analysis format of the ECG rhythm strips.

1.9.22 Describe two common methods for calculating heart rate on a ECG rhythm strip and the indications for using each method.

1.9.23 Name 8 causes of dysrhythmias.

S1.9.24 Demonstrate on an adult mannequin the techniques for single and two-person CPR according to American Heart Association standards.

S1.9.25 Demonstrate on an infant mannequin the technique for infant CPR according to American Heart Association standards.

S1.9.26 Demonstrate proper application of ECG chest electrodes and obtain a sample Lead II.

S1.9.27 Demonstrate the proper use of the defibrillator paddles electrodes to obtain a sample Lead II rhythm strip.

S1.9.28 Demonstrate how to properly assess the cause of poor ECG tracing.

S1.9.29 Demonstrate correct operation of a monitor-defibrillator to perform defibrillation on an adult and infant.

Index